Spiritual Care
in Practice

Spiritual Care
in Practice

Case Studies in Healthcare Chaplaincy

Edited by George Fitchett and Steve Nolan

Foreword by Christina M. Puchalski
Afterword by John Swinton

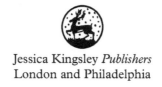

Jessica Kingsley *Publishers*
London and Philadelphia

First published in 2015
by Jessica Kingsley Publishers
73 Collier Street
London N1 9BE, UK
and
400 Market Street, Suite 400
Philadelphia, PA 19106, USA

www.jkp.com

Library of Congress Cataloging in Publication Data
Spiritual care in practice : case studies in healthcare chaplaincy
/ edited by George Fitchett and Steve Nolan.
p. ; cm.
Includes bibliographical references.
ISBN 978-1-84905-976-3
I. Fitchett, George, 1948- , editor. II. Nolan, Steve, editor.
[DNLM: 1. Pastoral Care--methods. 2. Chaplaincy Service,
Hospital--methods. 3. Patients--psychology.
4. Spirituality. WM 61]
BL65.M4
259'.42--dc23
2014028469

British Library Cataloguing in Publication Data
A CIP catalogue record for this book is available from the British Library

ISBN 978 1 84905 976 3
eISBN 978 0 85700 876 3

Printed and bound in Great Britain

Contents

Part 4   Ethical Concerns

Foreword

Christina M. Puchalski

'What is a chaplain?' 'How is a chaplain different from a counselor?' 'What do chaplains do?' These are the types of questions I hear from my colleagues as I speak about the importance of interprofessional spiritual care. And that is usually when I say, how is it possible not to work with chaplains in every facet of healthcare – inpatient, outpatient, clinician education and community health centers? What usually underlies these questions is the need for non-chaplain clinicians to learn more about the profession of chaplaincy. What better way to do this than through cases that demonstrate the richness of spiritual care and the power of the chaplain – an essential member of the healthcare team.

I have had the privilege to work with chaplains in a variety of settings – in the hospital, in our outpatient palliative care clinic at the George Washington University Medical Faculty Associates and in our medical schools, where trained chaplains co-mentor professional development sessions. In all of those settings, I see the power of the narrative approach in the evolving relationship between the chaplain and the patient or the student or the clinician. In this approach the patient's story unfolds within the relationship with the chaplain. Art Lucas called this the 'confluence of narrative' – 'As one journeys, hunkers down, is fully present with another' (Lucas 2008). Indeed, is this not also the process for all of us who journey with those whom we serve?

Fitchett and Canada's (2010) definition of chaplaincy assessment is that out of the patient narrative, which is shared in the relationship, the chaplain is able to develop a spiritual care plan with specific outcomes that is then communicated to the team. Some might call this a medicalization of spiritual care, but I see this as placing the patient's spiritual needs at the heart of medical care, at the heart of the reductionist medical model. This clinical partnership between healthcare professionals and chaplains is resulting in a transformation of this model. In a strictly medical model patients get labeled as 'the diabetic', 'the colon cancer', and so forth, resulting in the loss of the whole story of the patient. Chaplains don't label. They listen intently to the person – what they believe and what they value most. Working side by side with chaplains empowers the rest of the clinical team to see the whole person, to hear their story and to be fully present to the suffering of their patient.

Fitchett and Nolan's collection of chaplain case studies demonstrates the essential role of chaplains in clinical care. The cases demonstrate the importance of spiritual issues in clinical care and what the chaplain does in identifying and addressing patients' spiritual issues. The cases challenge chaplains to develop theories for chaplains as well as be leaders in clinical research in spiritual care, in quality improvement projects, in education of physicians, nurses and others, and in health policy. But the cases also educate other healthcare professionals about chaplaincy and also how patients' spiritual issues present in care, leading to a greater awareness of the spiritual needs of patients.

References

Fitchett, G. and Canada, A.L. (2010) 'The role of religion/spirituality in coping with cancer: Evidence, assessment and intervention.' In J. Holland, W. Breitbart, P. Jacobsen, M. Lederberg, M. Loscalzo and R. McCorkle (eds) *Psycho-oncology* (2nd edn.). New York, NY: Oxford University Press, 440–446.

Lucas, A. (2008) Presentation to Association of Professional Chaplains, Annual Meeting, Pittsburg, PA.

Introduction

George Fitchett

The case for chaplain case studies

This is a book of case studies about the work that healthcare chaplains do. We created this book because we believe developing a robust body of case studies is crucial at this point in the history of healthcare chaplains. Case study is a term that is used to refer to quite a range of research methods including studies of individuals, groups and organizations (Brown 2010; Yin 2014). These different methods of case study research are used by investigators from many disciplines including psychotherapists, sociologists, educators, economists and community planners. Some case studies are based on more than one case. While many case studies fall in the category of qualitative research, other case studies, including one chaplain case study (Risk 2013), have a quantitative component. In this book, case study refers to an in-depth report of a healthcare chaplain's care for a patient, and/or their family and friends, and the chaplain's critical reflections on that care.

There is growing recognition among chaplains around the world that we need to be a research-informed profession, both in order to examine and improve the care we provide and to help us describe the benefits of our care to our healthcare colleagues and the people responsible for commissioning our care. However, to conduct a study of the impact of chaplains' care, for example, a study to examine the effect of chaplains' care on the quality of life of patients with advanced cancer in palliative care, we need to know what it is that chaplains usually do with such patients. At present, we have very little published information about what chaplains do and, consequently, we would have problems developing such a study. Having five or ten published case studies of chaplains' work with advanced cancer patients would provide information about the salient components of the chaplain's care. Knowing those components, we could then design a study to test whether a chaplain's spiritual care had any effect on important outcomes, such as spiritual distress or quality of life of those patients. Case studies can provide an important foundation for the research chaplains need to do.[1]

Case studies can also play an important role in training new chaplains and in the continuing education of experienced chaplains. In countries such as the US, where clinical pastoral education (CPE) programs play a key role in their training, new chaplains mostly learn from cases written by the least experienced members of our profession, the cases they and their peers share in their CPE programs. A body of case studies written by experienced chaplains would deepen the learning of chaplains in training. Those who teach chaplains, including CPE supervisors, could lead discussions of published case studies as a way to teach chaplains in training how to think critically about the care provided and, by extension, the spiritual care they provide. Case studies also have a role in the continuing education of experienced chaplains, who could use them to compare perspectives about best practices in specific clinical situations.

Finally, case studies can play a critical role in helping colleagues in other health professions develop a better understanding of what chaplains do. As most chaplains know, despite efforts to increase courses in medical and nursing schools (Koenig *et al.* 2010), very few of our colleagues in medicine or nursing or other health professions receive substantive training about the spiritual dimension of health or the role of the chaplain in the healthcare team (Balboni *et al.* 2013; Rasinski *et al.* 2011). Giving colleagues a published case study is an effective way to help them better understand the work that we do. Because case studies can be emotionally engaging, they are also an effective method for educating healthcare decision makers and the public about the work that chaplains do.

What case studies have chaplains published?

Despite the importance of case studies for our profession, the chaplain case study literature is very limited. As Folland (2006) says, 'At the moment precious little is known about what happens when chaplain and patient meet' (p.17). This is somewhat surprising given the central role of case studies in the work of Anton Boisen, a leader in the development of CPE and modern chaplaincy in the US. Boisen had an intense interest in case studies (Asquith 1980, 1990). He is best remembered for *Out of the Depths* (Boisen 1960), his case study about his own experience with mental illness. However, throughout his career he was writing case studies and examining patterns in these cases as a way to better understand the relationship between religion and mental illness. Students in his CPE programs spent their time reading and discussing the cases Boisen wrote (Boisen 1971).[2] Boisen's interest in case studies was not sustained by other early chaplaincy leaders. In fact, just as Boisen's book about his case study research was being published (1936/1971), Cabot and Dicks' influential volume, *The Art of Ministering to the Sick*, appeared (1936). It included Chaplain Russell Dicks' chapter encouraging chaplains to make 'note-writing' a regular practice. The impact of Dicks' work contributed to case studies being replaced by verbatims in the early CPE programs in the US (Hall 1992; Holifield 1990; King 2007). Since then, verbatims have remained the predominant method used to facilitate reflection on the conversations between chaplains and patients.

In searching the chaplaincy literature prior to 2011, I have not found any published case studies in the sense that we use the term in this book, an in-depth report of a chaplain's care and their critical reflections on that care. (I am happy to have readers point out any cases I may have missed.) Our literature does contain articles and book chapters that include case studies, and some have the term 'case study' in the titles (Berger 2001; Gibbons and Miller 1989; Isgandarova 2008; Pervis-Smith 1996); however, these texts were usually written to illustrate one or more points about a chaplain's care, and the case reports are generally brief. I have found examples of extended reports of a chaplain's care, but they did not include the chaplain's critical reflection (Gibbons 1988). In my work on spiritual assessment, I have also published five case studies (Fitchett 1993, 1995; Fitchett and Roberts 2003). Each of these cases was written to illustrate the 7×7 model for spiritual assessment. As such, they give detailed information about the patients in the cases, especially my spiritual assessment of them, but they do not include detailed information about the spiritual care provided nor the outcomes of the cases.[3]

An important, brief case study deserves recognition. In what may be the first paper to use the term 'evidence-based pastoral care', O'Connor and Meakes (1998) describe the case of Mary, a 40-year-old woman with cerebral palsy, who lived in a chronic care hospital. After the onset of seizure activity, Mary was no longer able to use her electric wheelchair. This left her feeling depressed, unable to attend church as she had in the past, and wondering why God would not help her. This brief case description (one paragraph) is followed by a review of research that would be relevant to providing spiritual care for Mary, including research about spirituality and disability. As the authors note, at the time there was actually very little research that was directly relevant to this case. After this literature review, the authors describe the spiritual care provided to Mary and the changes that occurred as a result of that care. While brief, these descriptions include a remarkable level of specificity about the counseling interventions that took place.

The absence of published chaplain case studies stands in contrast to psychotherapy where there are journals devoted to cases (e.g. *Pragmatic Case Studies in Psychotherapy*), books of case studies (e.g. Goldberg

1978), including books about integrating spirituality in psychotherapy (Richards and Bergin 2004), and databases of cases designed to advance case study research (Miller 2004; see also the website for *Pragmatic Case Studies in Psychotherapy*[4]). As chaplains work to develop a body of case studies there is much we can learn from the work in these related fields.

The year 2011 saw the publication of the first chaplain case study as we use the term here. In that year, Rhonda Cooper published a description of her work with a woman with advanced breast cancer who was afraid about dying (Cooper 2011). This case study grew out of a group of oncology chaplains I recruited to write case studies about their work (Fitchett 2011), and it was followed by one from Stephen King, who described his work with a woman with leukemia (King 2012). Because it is important not only to publish case studies about our work but to engage in critical discussion about them, both of these cases were accompanied by commentary from other chaplains (King 2011; Maddox 2012) as well as from colleagues in health psychology (Canada 2011) and pastoral counseling (Schlauch 2012). More recently, my colleague Jay Risk published a case study of his work with a patient whose sense of meaning in life was shattered by Parkinson's disease (Risk 2013). Responses to Risk's case included a chaplain (Grossoehme 2013), a pastoral counselor (Giblin 2013) and a health psychologist (Emery 2013). These three cases studies, and their related commentaries, provide a helpful start for building a body of case studies for our field.

Creating this book of chaplain case studies

Steve Nolan and I created this book to build on this beginning. To find the cases for this book, we sent invitations to contribute a case study to chaplaincy associations, groups of chaplains and individual chaplains whom we knew around the world (UK, US, Canada, Europe, Australia and Israel). We stipulated that contributors needed to have at least 3 years' of experience in healthcare chaplaincy, and we asked those who were interested to submit an 800-word summary of their case. Based on these submissions, we invited nine chaplains to contribute the cases in this book. The criteria that guided our selection of these cases included: a desire for cases from chaplains working in different national contexts; for diversity in the religious traditions of the chaplains and patients/ families; and for cases that illustrated common or important issues in chaplaincy practice. It ended up that we had three groups of case studies, with three cases each from chaplains working in pediatrics, psychiatry and palliative care.

In developing their case studies for this book we asked the chaplains to address three things: the first was to give the context for the case, that is, to provide information about the patient (and/or family), about themselves and their institutional context; the second was to describe the history of the chaplain-patient relationship, focusing on significant moments and interventions in the relationship, and including verbatim accounts of important conversations, if they were available; the third was to step back from the case and describe and critically reflect on their assessment of the patient, their interventions and the changes that did or did not occur as a result of the care they provided (outcomes). The aim of this outline was to provide you with the information you need to put yourself in the chaplain's shoes and to think about how the care you would provide for this patient would be similar to or different from that provided by the author of the case.[5]

Beginning a conversation

In publishing these case studies, one of our central aims has been to promote a conversation about the work that chaplains do. As such, we not only recruited these case studies but also recruited respondents who would read the cases and begin a conversation about them. For each of the three groups of cases we recruited two respondents: the first respondent is an experienced chaplain, who has worked in the area from which the cases come; the second is a colleague from another healthcare profession (psychology, nursing or medicine), who again has experience in that clinical area.

We asked the respondents to focus their critical reflection on two things: first, on the care the chaplains reported providing; this included how the chaplains' care contributed to the patients' well-being or recovery, opportunities for care that the chaplains may have missed or care which seemed inappropriate. Second, we asked the respondents to examine how the chaplains reflected on their care, on key concepts the chaplains employed or overlooked as they wrote about their assessments, interventions and outcomes. We also welcomed the respondents' thoughts about what case studies such as these could contribute to chaplaincy, as well as any reflections about chaplaincy and healthcare. To further the conversation we also invited Professor John Swinton to review the whole volume and share his thoughts about what case studies such as these can contribute to chaplaincy, as well as his reflections about chaplaincy and healthcare.

In selecting these cases, there are two things we don't wish to communicate. We don't wish readers, especially readers unfamiliar with healthcare chaplaincy, to think of these cases as representative of what *most* chaplains do. There are elements in each of the cases, such as listening, or offering comfort, guidance and hospitality, that will feel very familiar to most chaplains; however, the cases were not selected to provide a picture of the average chaplain's day or week. Furthermore, while we think in each case the chaplain's care had positive effects on these patients and families, we don't claim that the cases are examples of ideal chaplaincy care. We see strengths and weaknesses in each of them and we are sure you will too. As such, we think the case studies in this book provide a good place to begin a conversation about what chaplains do.

Let me contribute to that conversation by sharing a few of my thoughts about the cases. One of the first things that strikes me about them is diversity; diversity in their clinical contexts for sure, but also diversity in the religious and cultural background of the patients and families. They are also diverse in the length of time over which the chaplain-patient relationships extended, from 1 day to several weeks to several years. Because chaplains often speak of the challenges of providing care in acute-care settings, where patient stays are so short, the multi-year relationships described in the cases by Chaplains Huth and Roberts and Chaplain Hildebrand are quite striking. The cases are also diverse in how long ago they occurred. Chaplain Grossoehme describes a case that is ongoing. The cases from Chaplains Huth and Roberts and Chaplain Zollfrank are relatively recent. In contrast, several of the cases took place years ago (the cases by Ratcliffe, Piderman, Redl), and in one case (Swift), several decades ago.

The key themes in the cases are also diverse. In several cases, engaging cultural difference with hospitality and respect is central (Weyls, Ratcliffe). Rituals play an important role in the majority of the cases (Grossoehme, Hildebrand, Zollfrank, Swift, Redl, Huth and Roberts), and in one case they are central (Weyls). In a number of the cases the chaplain provides guidance, helping to address uncertainty about treatment decisions (Huth and Roberts) or conflicts related to religious beliefs (Piderman, Zollfrank, Swift). In several cases, what stands out is how the chaplain provided sustaining support in the face of long illness with an uncertain course (Grossoehme, Hildebrand), or sensitive listening that relieved suffering at the end of life (Redl).

What was it about each of these relationships that led our contributors to share their case? Our relationships with some patients touch us deeply; something about the patient's suffering, their grace, the positive impact of our care, our uncertainty about what we did or didn't do.[6] Writing about their cases seems like it has been a way for these chaplains to share an important lesson learned about this work, to explore what did and didn't happen in the relationship, to make an argument about what chaplains do, to memorialize a beloved patient.

Next steps in chaplain case studies

It is our hope that the nine cases in this book will be followed by the publication of many more chaplain case studies and critical responses to those case studies from chaplains and other healthcare colleagues. For our profession to realize the full benefit of case studies that I described earlier, many chaplains need to get involved in writing and publishing their cases and in engaging in critical discussion of one another's work. As we build this body of case studies there are important ethical issues to keep in mind, including whether to obtain permission to publish from the subject of the case and how to protect their confidentiality. In each of the case studies in this book, the chaplains describe how they addressed these issues. Because it is essential to be attentive to these issues, we have included a helpful chapter on ethical issues in case study research by David McCurdy.

Let me conclude this Introduction with several recommendations. We should encourage workshops about case studies in local, regional and national chaplaincy conferences. These could include beginning workshops about how to write case studies, as well as more advanced workshops where experienced chaplains discuss the strengths and weaknesses of one or more case studies. In addition, we should encourage the publication of case studies in chaplaincy journals. To advance our field it is especially important for some of those case studies to be accompanied by the kind of critical responses that are included in this book. As we do this we need to expand the kinds of cases we present and publish to include mundane cases and the cases that didn't go well, along with those that went very well. We also need cases from clinical contexts beyond those represented in this book.

In addition to what we do within our profession, it is important for chaplains to share their cases with healthcare colleagues in other professions, at their grand rounds, in-services, conferences and in their journals. The importance of this was underscored by the comment of a chaplain who participated in a study about chaplains and quality improvement: '[A colleague] and I did a presentation to a palliative care conference… And what we did was [role play] a verbatim… We brought down the house because it was like they never…experienced a chaplain's visit before' (Lyndes *et al.* 2008, p.74). The majority of our healthcare colleagues have little or no education to help them gain a meaningful appreciation for what we contribute to the care of patients and their families. This isn't going to change quickly, so chaplains must be persistent and creative in looking for ways to tell the story of who we are and what we do. Case studies presented at the professional meetings of other health professions and published in the journals that our healthcare colleagues read, perhaps with a discussion of the case by a colleague from that discipline, would be a very effective use of case studies to educate our colleagues about our work.

Summary and acknowledgements

Case studies were central to the work of Anton Boisen, a founder of modern chaplaincy and CPE in the US. They play a central role in developing the foundation for research about the effects of chaplains' spiritual care. They can also be an effective way to help colleagues in other healthcare professions develop a better understanding of the chaplains' contribution to care for patients and families. Healthcare chaplaincy is in the process of becoming a research-informed profession. Many chaplains can play an important role in this process, not by conducting randomized clinical trials or other quantitative research, but by writing case studies about the work they do every day.

We would not have been able to begin this conversation about what chaplains do without the contributions of the nine chaplains who share their cases in this book. It is not often that practicing chaplains share the details of their work for critical review by their colleagues, and it takes some courage to do that. Beyond that, several of these chaplains shared drafts of their cases with the patients/families about whom they were writing, a type of feedback that is even less common for us. We acknowledge our deep appreciation to these chaplains for letting us share their work with you. We also acknowledge our gratitude to the patients and families whose stories are in these case studies.

Endnotes

1   Many readers will know that the levels of evidence hierarchies commonly employed for evaluating medical research assign a low rank to evidence from case studies (Straus *et al.* 2011). There is sound reasoning behind these hierarchies. At the same time, the important information that can be obtained from case study research should not be underestimated. Yin (2014) provides an excellent response to critics who see only the limitations of case study research. Also see the excellent article by Flyvbjerg (2006).

2   More than 30 of Boisen's cases, as well as a copy of his 13-page case study outline, can be viewed at a website created by Boisen scholar Jesús Rodríguez Sánchez at the Interamerican University of Puerto Rico (see www.metro.inter.edu/facultad/esthumanisticos/anton_boisen.htm, accessed on 4 July 2014).

3   While the chaplaincy case study literature is not well developed, there is a literature about the use of case studies in field education and ministry formation (e.g. Mahan, Troxell and Allen 1993; Northcott 2000). For an overview of case studies in practical theology see Schipani (2012).

4   http://pcsp.libraries.rutgers.edu/index.php/pcsp/about/pcspAbout, accessed on 4 July 2014.

5   Elsewhere (Fitchett 2011), I have described another outline for the contents of a good case study, based in part on the important work on case studies by the psychologist Ron Miller (2004). For other outlines see the Instructions to Authors for *Pragmatic Case Studies in Psychotherapy* (pcsp.libraries.rutgers.edu/index.php/pcsp/about/pcspAuthorInstructions, accessed on 4 July 2014) and *Clinical Case Studies* (www.sagepub.com/journals/Journal201493/manuscriptSubmission, accessed on 4 July 2014).

6   This also seems to have been the case for Russell Dicks. See the four cases he included in Appendix A (Cabot and Dicks 1936), and especially his description of the impact on him of caring for JL, a young woman with an inoperable cancer (Cabot and Dicks 1936, pp.359–371).

References

Asquith, G.H. Jr. (1980) 'The case study method of Anton T. Boisen.' *Journal of Pastoral Care 34*, 2, 84–94.

Asquith, G.H. Jr. (1990) 'Case study method.' In R.J. Hunter (ed) *Dictionary of Pastoral Care and Counseling*. Nashville, TN: Abingdon Press, 123–126.

Balboni, M.J., Sullivan, A., Amobi, A., Phelps, A.C. *et al.* (2013) 'Why is spiritual care infrequent at the end of life? Spiritual care perceptions among patients, nurses, and physicians and the role of training.' *Journal of Clinical Oncology 31*, 4, 461–467.

Berger, J.A. (2001) 'A case study: Linda.' *Journal of Health Care Chaplaincy 10*, 2, 35–43. Co-published as L. VandeCreek and A.M. Lucas (eds) (2001) *The Discipline for Pastoral Care Giving*. Binghamton, NY: The Haworth Pastoral Press, 35–43.

Boisen, A.T. (1960) *Out of the Depths: An Autobiographical Study of Mental Disorder and Religious Experience*. New York, NY: Harper & Brothers.

Boisen, A.T. (1971) *The Exploration of the Inner World: A Study of Mental Disorder and Religious Experience*. Philadelphia, PA: University of Pennsylvania Press. (Original work published 1936.)

Brown, L. (2010) 'Making the case for case study research.' *Chaplaincy Today 26*, 2, 2–15.

Cabot, R.C. and Dicks, R.L. (1936) *The Art of Ministering to the Sick*. New York, NY: Macmillan.

Canada, A.L. (2011) 'A psychologist's response to the case study: Application of theory and measurement.' *Journal of Health Care Chaplaincy 17*, 1–2, 46–54.

Cooper, R.S. (2011) 'Case study of a chaplain's spiritual care for a patient with advanced metastatic breast cancer.' *Journal of Health Care Chaplaincy 17*, 1–2, 19–37.

Emery, E.E. (2013) 'Who am I with Parkinson's disease? A psychologist response to chaplain intervention in the context of identity theory.' *Journal of Health Care Chaplaincy 19*, 3, 120–129.

Fitchett, G. (1993) *Assessing Spiritual Needs: A Guide for Caregivers*. Minneapolis, MN: Augsburg Fortress.

Fitchett, G. (1995) 'Linda Krauss and the lap of God: A spiritual assessment case study.' *Second Opinion 20*, 4, 41–49.

Fitchett, G. (2011) 'Making our case(s).' *Journal of Health Care Chaplaincy 17*, 1–2, 3–18.

Fitchett, G. and Roberts, P.A. (2003) 'In the garden with Andrea: Spiritual assessment in end of life care.' In C.M. Puchalski (ed) *Walking Together: Physicians, Chaplains and Clergy Caring for the Sick*. Washington, DC: The George Washington Institute for Spirituality and Health, 23–31.

Flyvbjerg, B. (2006) 'Five misunderstandings about case-study research.' *Qualitative Inquiry 12*, 2, 219–245.

Folland, M. (2006) 'Opportunity and conflict: Evidence-based practice and the modernization of healthcare chaplaincy.' *Contact 149*, 12–20.

Gibbons, G.D. (1988) 'Embodiment: ministry, sacrament and evangelism: A case study.' *Ministry, Society and Theology 2*, 2, 1–11.

Gibbons, J.L. and Miller, S.L. (1989) 'An image of contemporary hospital chaplaincy.' *Journal of Pastoral Care 43*, 4, 355–361.

Giblin, P. (2013) 'Building a new life: A pastoral counselor's response.' *Journal of Health Care Chaplaincy 19*, 3, 112–119.

Goldberg, A. (ed) (1978) *The Psychology of the Self: A Casebook*. New York, NY: International Universities Press.

Grossoehme, D.H. (2013) 'Chaplaincy and narrative theory: A response to Risk's case study.' *Journal of Health Care Chaplaincy 19*, 3, 99–111.

Hall, C.E. (1992) *Head and Heart: The Story of the Clinical Pastoral Education Movement*. Decatur, GA: Journal of Pastoral Care Publications.

Holifield, E.B. (1990) 'Dicks, Russell.' In R.J. Hunter (ed) *Dictionary of Pastoral Care and Counseling*. Nashville, TN: Abingdon Press, 284.

Isgandarova, N. (2008) 'Muslim spiritual care and counseling: A case study of a resident with Parkinson's disease.' In T.S. O'Connor, C. Lashmar and E. Meakes (eds) *The Spiritual Care Giver's Guide to Identity, Practice and Relationships: Transforming the Honeymoon in Spiritual Care and Therapy*. Halifax, NS: South Western Region of the Canadian Association for Pastoral Practice and Education and Waterloo, ON: Waterloo Lutheran Seminary, 235–242.

King, S.D.W. (2007) *Trust the Process: A History of Clinical Pastoral Education as Theological Education*. Lanham, MD: University Press of America.

King, S.D.W. (2011) 'Touched by an angel: A chaplain's response to the case study's key interventions, styles, and themes/outcomes.' *Journal of Health Care Chaplaincy 17*, 1–2, 38–45.

King, S.D.W. (2012). 'Facing fears and counting blessings: A case study of a chaplain's faithful companioning a cancer patient.' *Journal of Health Care Chaplaincy 18*, 1–2, 3–22.

Koenig, H.G., Hooten, E.G., Lindsay-Calkins, E. and Meador, K.G. (2010) 'Spirituality in medical school curricula: Findings from a national survey.' *International Journal of Psychiatry Medicine 40*, 4, 391–398.

Lyndes, K.A., Fitchett, G., Thomason, C.L., Berlinger, N. and Jacobs, M.R. (2008) 'Chaplains and quality improvement: Can we make our case by improving our care?' *Journal of Health Care Chaplaincy 15*, 2, 65–79.

Maddox, R.T. (2012) 'The chaplain as faithful companion: A response to King's case study.' *Journal of Health Care Chaplaincy 18*, 1–2, 33–42.

Mahan, J.H., Troxell, B.B. and Allen, C.J. (1993) *Shared Wisdom: A Guide to Case Study Reflection in Ministry*. Nashville, TN: Abingdon Press.

Miller, R.B. (2004) *Facing Human Suffering: Psychology and Psychotherapy as Moral Engagement*. Washington, DC: American Psychological Association.

Northcott, M. (2000) 'The case study method in theological education.' In D. Willows and J. Swinton (eds) *Spiritual Dimensions of Pastoral Care*. London: Jessica Kingsley Publishers, 59–65.

O'Connor, T.S. and Meakes, E. (1998) 'Hope in the midst of challenge: Evidence-based pastoral care.' *Journal of Pastoral Care 52*, 4, 359–367.

Pervis-Smith, T.A. (1996) 'Pediatric pastoral care: A case study.' *Journal of Pastoral Care 50*, 2, 171–180.

Rasinski, K.A., Kalad, Y.G., Yoon, J.D. and Curlin, F.A. (2011) 'An assessment of US physicians' training in religion, spirituality, and medicine.' *Medical Teacher 33*, 11, 944–945.

Richards, P.S. and Bergin, A.E. (eds) (2004) *Casebook for a Spiritual Strategy in Counseling and Psychotherapy*. Washington, DC: American Psychological Association.

Risk, J.L. (2013) 'Building a new life: A chaplain's theory based case study of chronic illness.' *Journal of Health Care Chaplaincy 19*, 3, 81–98.

Schipani, D.S. (2012) 'Case study method.' In B. Miller-McLemore (ed) *The Wiley-Blackwell Companion to Practical Theology*. Chichester: John Wiley and Sons, 91–101.

Schlauch, C.R. (2012) 'A pastoral theologian's response to the case study.' *Journal of Health Care Chaplains 18*, 1–2, 23–32.

Straus, S.E., Glasziou, P., Richardson, W.S., Haynes, R.B. (2011) *Evidence-based Medicine: How to Practice and Teach It* (4th edn). Edinburgh: Churchill Livingstone and Elsevier.

Yin, R.K. (2014) *Case Study Research: Design and Methods* (5th edn). Thousand Oaks, CA: Sage Publications.

Part I
Pediatric Case Studies

Steve Nolan

The three case studies that follow detail work that is typical of chaplains active in pediatric care. As the first writer makes clear, chaplaincy in pediatric healthcare differs from that of adult healthcare in that it needs to be informed by an understanding of child development (Smith and McSherry 2004). At the very least, this makes the already uncertain territory of assessing spiritual needs more complex. But it also means that chaplains in this area must tailor their interventions to be appropriate to the child's developmental stage. Such interventions are likely to require a higher degree of creativity than those in adult healthcare: storytelling or imaginative play (Hufton 2006), for example, or drawing and painting, as is demonstrated in our first case.

In relating an account of his work with LeeAnn, a 12-year-old girl with cystic fibrosis, Chaplain Grossoehme describes work that is typical of his spiritual care approach to children living with chronic illness. This work aims, of course, to give spiritual support in the present moment, but equally it has, as a key aspect, a forward-looking focus in that it aims at building and maintaining a long-term relationship, knowing that one day LeeAnn or her family may need an honest and open discussion of religious or existential questions with a trusted spiritual advisor.

To that end, Chaplain Grossoehme demonstrates how chaplaincy practice can be informed and directed by a narrative approach derived from Kleinman's (1988) account of three archetypal narratives: *chaos* narratives, which lurch from crisis to crisis; *restitution* narratives, which speak of a return to life the way it was before; or *quest* narratives, which seek to learn from an event, however awful. Having first established a relationship with LeeAnn, Chaplain Grossoehme encourages her to narrate her story, which he identifies as a restitution narrative. This suggests to him that he should focus on building a relationship with LeeAnn, and also on integrating her 'secular' interests of drawing and playing with the sacred dimension of her life. To that end, he shows how he enabled LeeAnn to describe her relationship with God through drawing and how he extended this by encouraging her to use drawing as a means of prayer.

Chaplain Grossoehme notes that a critical element of narrative theory is that listening to a story impacts the listener. He relates something of his self-reflection as people speak to him about his work. But in relating LeeAnn's experience of living with cystic fibrosis and the burdensome regime of daily treatment, Chaplain Grossoehme also highlights the way in which hospital treatment imposed a necessary, but additional, isolation on LeeAnn that also impacted on the way he was able to deliver spiritual care. Being compliant with infection guidelines meant that Chaplain Grossoehme was required to wear a paper gown, face mask and gloves during his encounters with LeeAnn. This physical barrier not only reinforced a whole series of differences that existed between Chaplain Grossoehme, as the chaplain, and LeeAnn, as the person who was sick, but also interfered with normal facial and non-verbal communication, denaturalizing and depersonalizing the encounter. Perhaps in part to compensate for these additional barriers, Chaplain Grossoehme describes using a particular question intended to pique interest and foster reflective conversation. He has found this question works well with adolescents, and the follow-up discussion enables him to explore their answers further.

The impact of spiritual care on the chaplain comes across clearly in the case study presented by Chaplain Hildebrand. She describes her work with Erica, a young mother of a 2-year-old girl with cancer, work that had a very personal involvement. Chaplain Hildebrand became aware that, while Erica had a keen Christian faith, she shared nothing of this with the hospital social workers. Equally, while she appeared to trust Chaplain Hildebrand, there were aspects of her life, specifically details of her family, which Erica seemed not to want to share with Chaplain Hildebrand. Erica was controlling which aspects of her story she told to which professionals, possibly on the basis that different professionals would be able to accept different aspects of her lifestyle and not judge her for those aspects. Chaplain Hildebrand's study models good practice in multi-professional working in that sharing of relevant information between professionals enabled her to make a contribution specific to her role as a chaplain, which, in this case, is related to the chaplain's ability to enter the world of another person's belief system and engage them with the kind of empathic understanding that is simultaneously objective *and* subjective. In terms of Christian theology, this case models an incarnational approach.

The study also illustrates the role intuition can play in good spiritual care, particularly when it is informed by experience and multi-professional liaison. Sensing that Erica was censoring her involvement in substance abuse, Chaplain Hildebrand demonstrates how judicious self-disclosure can deepen spiritual care work with some people. Self-disclosure is a sensitive subject within the counselling literature and, depending on orientation, counsellor-therapists either abjure all self-disclosure or recognize its place and work carefully with it (see Clarkson 2003, pp.160–167). But, while humanistic counsellor-therapists will acknowledge that, wisely used, self-disclosure 'has potential to promote positive change and to assist in the development of a good therapeutic alliance. Clearly, though, doing it well requires good clinical judgment and attunement to clients' needs' (Bloomgarden and Mennuti 2009, p.3), there is little guidance for chaplains, either on the value and efficacy of self-disclosure or on its proper use. Among therapist researchers, self-disclosure is acknowledged as an inevitable and unavoidable aspect of psychotherapy: therapists constantly 'give themselves away' (Wosket

1999, p.51). However, therapist researchers also note an important ethical difficulty with self-disclosure in that it can be a first step towards violating the boundaries of the therapeutic relationship (Barnett 1998). Barnett (2011) recommends that therapists thoughtfully consider their motivations, the treatment needs and personal history of their clients and the differences that exist between themselves and their client. In self-disclosing to Erica, Chaplain Hildebrand demonstrates Barnett's (2011) recommendations and offers chaplains an example of good practice in this sensitive area.

In her study, Chaplain Piderman presents another example of a chaplain empathically entering another person's world view, in this case to work therapeutically with their beliefs. In engaging 17-year-old Angela, paralyzed by injuries sustained in a car accident, Chaplain Piderman found an adolescent buoyed initially by her mother's assertions that 'God never gives you more than you can take' and 'If you pray hard enough, God will give you a miracle'; but who later experienced profound emotional and spiritual despair by God's apparent absence. In this situation, Chaplain Piderman states one of her goals was 'to be a sign of God's incarnational love' – making explicit what is implied in this case – by 'remaining present' and entering Angela's darkness, sustaining herself by keeping her eyes on the light of hope.

Chaplain Piderman records how her work with Angela posed for her the difficult question of whether to challenge beliefs she regarded as unhelpful, if not unhealthy, and, if so, *how* to challenge them. This is a difficulty chaplains frequently face that calls for high levels of personal awareness and theological skill. To make an ill-judged challenge could irretrievably damage the chaplain's relationship with the person they are aiming to help; equally, it could be ethically inappropriate. In detailing her motivations, step by step, Chaplain Piderman makes clear what she wanted to achieve and what she felt were the risks both if she challenged Angela or if she declined to challenge her. Chaplain Piderman's skill is such that she models how another person's unhealthy beliefs might be challenged, with respect and compassion and in a way that opens an opportunity for healing. In so doing, she gives an account of the pastoral imperative associated with the problem of theodicy: how to reconcile suffering with the idea that God is *both* all-loving and all-powerful.

Clearly, this intensive work with Angela had its impact on Chaplain Piderman, and she ends her study with a brief but helpful reflection on her feelings when it came time for Angela to be discharged. Here Chaplain Piderman draws attention to the value of boundaries for a chaplain's self-care.

The chaplain respondent to these cases, Alister W. Bull, has conducted doctoral research concerned with developing a tool to assess the spiritual needs of children in hospital. Bull identifies some common themes threading through the studies; in particular, he highlights the theoretical frameworks chaplains use to reflect upon their visits. These frameworks are often implicit and may even be unrecognized by chaplains. The reader may find it interesting to compare these implied frameworks with Richard C. Weyls' explicit theoretical framework in the final case (Chapter 13) – what he calls his 'operative theology of spiritual care'. Bull also draws attention to a phenomenon little discussed among chaplains: the place of pastoral power in chaplaincy encounters.

The related healthcare professional, Sian Cotton, is a clinical health psychologist and researcher in pediatric health outcomes research, with experience working closely with chaplains. Cotton considers each case in turn. She wonders whether Chaplain Grossoehme is correct to assert that relationship building can be an outcome in itself, and she is curious about why the topic of 'endings' was not raised more with a child who has a life-shortening condition. In relation to Chaplain Hildebrand, Cotton raises a question about models of chaplaincy care, and wonders whether the desire to go beyond religious conversation to a 'deeper level' is achievable in shorter-term, crisis-oriented models (a point also raised by Bull). She is also struck by Chaplain Hildebrand's goal of '[getting] religion out of the way so that spiritual care could begin', and she wonders about her definition of 'spiritual care'. Finally, with Chaplain Piderman, Cotton highlights an important practice-based research opportunity and the important role chaplains can play within interdisciplinary teams.

References

Barnett, J.E. (1998) 'Should psychotherapists self-disclose? Clinical and ethical considerations.' In L. VandeCreek, S. Knapp and T.L. Jackson (eds) *Innovations in Clinical Practice: A Source Book 16*. Sarasota, FL: Professional Resource Press/ Professional Resource Exchange, 419–428.

Barnett, J.E. (2011) 'Psychotherapist self-disclosure: Ethical and clinical considerations.' *Psychotherapy: Theory, Research, Practice, Training 48*, 4, 315–321.

Bloomgarden, A. and Mennuti, R.B. (2009) 'Therapist self-disclosure: Beyond the taboo.' In A. Bloomgarden and R.B. Mennuti (eds) *Psychotherapist Revealed: Therapists Speak about Self-Disclosure in Psychotherapy*. New York, NY: Routledge, 3–16.

Clarkson, P. (2003) *The Therapeutic Relationship* (2nd edn). London: Whurr.

Hufton, E. (2006) 'Parting gifts: The spiritual needs of children.' *Journal of Child Health Care 10*, 3, 240–250.

Kleinman, A. (1988) *The Illness Narratives*. New York, NY: Basic Books.

Smith, J. and McSherry, W. (2004) 'Spirituality and child development: A concept analysis.' *Journal of Advanced Nursing 45*, 3, 307–315.

Wosket, V. (1999) *The Therapeutic Use of Self: Counselling Practice, Research and Supervision*. Hove: Brunner-Routledge.

Chapter 1

'God tells the doctors to pick the right medicine'

– LeeAnn, a 12-year-old girl with cystic fibrosis

Daniel H. Grossoehme

Introduction

This case study describes chaplaincy care over the course of approximately 1 year with LeeAnn (a pseudonym), a Euro-American girl who was then 12 years old. She is an only child who lives with her parents in a small community within 50 miles of Cincinnati, Ohio, a mid-sized city in the American Midwest. She attended seventh grade in her local (tax-funded) school, where she generally earned good grades. However, her school attendance had been poor; she missed 30–60 school days during the prior school year due to frequent hospitalizations and disease-related issues. LeeAnn is an engaging and social adolescent who enjoys activities typical for her age and gender: watching television, playing on the computer as well as singing. She had participated in cheerleading for her church's sports teams in the past. Her family are non-denominational Christians.

LeeAnn has cystic fibrosis (CF), which is a life-shortening genetic disease with a median life expectancy of approximately 37 years (US National Library of Medicine 2013). The genetic mutations of CF cause a failure of the body's sodium transport system in the cells, leading to an accumulation of mucus (Wilfond and Taussig 1999). While commonly considered a pulmonary disease, CF affects multiple organs, depending on what combination of the over 1500 mutations that cause CF a person actually has. In addition to the lungs, CF may affect the pancreas or liver; it may cause diabetes, sinusitis and nasal polyps, and sterility in males. The mucus layer must be cleared from the lungs to prevent infection; its coating of the intestinal walls prevents absorption of nutrients (Wilfond and Taussig 1999). Stringent infection control precautions strongly discourage in-person contact with other persons who have CF both while in and out of the hospital (Saiman *et al.* 2003). Persons with CF are generally not supposed to be within 6 feet of another person with the disease, the exception being other family members who have CF since maintaining such a distance is obviously not an option.

The daily home treatment regimen for persons with CF is burdensome and typically includes some form of airway clearance (chest physiotherapy) and inhalation of antibiotics or other drugs, which are aerosolized and inhaled through a face mask. Persons with CF may also require insulin (if diabetic) and nutritional enzymes before eating or drinking anything. The time required for all these treatments may range from 90 minutes to 2–3 hours per day. Not surprisingly, adherence to evidence-based treatment guidelines is typically less than 60% (Modi *et al.* 2006) and is both lower overall and more variable among adolescents (Ball *et al.* 2013; Bucks *et al.* 2009).

LeeAnn was diagnosed with CF in the first year of her life, and with CF-related diabetes between 4 and 5 years of age. She does well nutritionally and has a body mass index greater than the 50th percentile for her age and gender, consistent with CF Foundation guidelines (Stallings *et al.* 2008). During the year prior to this study, LeeAnn had been admitted to the hospital almost monthly for intravenous antibiotics and for a persistent cough. Over the course of her life, she has had multiple bronchoscopies and more than 100 surgeries, nearly all sinus surgeries to remove polyps associated with CF. Her pulmonologist was working with LeeAnn and her mother to prevent further hospitalizations or sinus surgeries by offering alternative drug therapies (inhaled antibiotics rather than intravenous); however, this was complicated by the fact that LeeAnn had developed resistance to most antibiotics. The pulmonologist and clinic staff were beginning to have discussions with LeeAnn and her mother about LeeAnn assuming an increased role in the self-management of her CF. LeeAnn's daily routine during this period began with waking before 5:00 a.m. to complete 30 minutes of airway clearance and to take her nebulized medications (with the assistance of her mother), a total of 60–90 minutes of morning care. She did not do any treatments while at school and repeated her morning routine in the evening.

I am an Episcopal priest and board certified chaplain (through the Association of Professional Chaplains), and I was 49 years old at the time of these encounters. I have been a pediatric hospital chaplain for 20 years. At present, approximately 25% of my effort is devoted to clinical chaplaincy, with the remaining 75% effort devoted to research. For the 5 years prior to these encounters, my clinical area has been the CF Center. The CF Center follows over 280 children and adolescents from a four-state region and is composed of an outpatient clinic, to which most patients come quarterly, and a 12-bed inpatient CF unit within our 523-bed academic pediatric medical center. At the time of this writing, most of my clinical work occurred on the inpatient unit. LeeAnn and I have been acquainted since I met her and her mother in the CF outpatient clinic 5 years ago and have seen each other intermittently in both inpatient and outpatient settings.

During the period of this case study, there were two chaplaincy issues. The first issue was that LeeAnn was frequently alone during the day while in hospital, as her mother was at work, though she was present evenings and weekends. At times, another family member stayed with LeeAnn. Related to being alone, there was another aspect to her isolation during her inpatient admissions. Infection guidelines for CF require all staff to don paper gowns, face masks and gloves before entering a patient room. While protecting people with CF from iatrogenic infections, they also form a physical barrier between the chaplain and the person, and make facial, non-verbal communication very difficult. The second chaplaincy issue was relationship building and maintenance. A focus of my care was to build and maintain a pastoral relationship with LeeAnn during her chronic, non-emergent hospitalizations so that she would feel free to ask religious/existential questions as she grew older and/or her disease progressed.

Case study
First encounter

Although I was acquainted with LeeAnn and her mother from previous meetings in the outpatient clinic, this was the first in a series of significant encounters on the inpatient unit. As such, my goals for this visit were to begin a narrative assessment process to determine whether follow-up care was indicated, and to build a relationship with LeeAnn for future encounters. LeeAnn engaged in a wide-ranging conversation with me. Commenting on a book on her bedside table about ghosts, our discussion moved to believing in ghosts, what it would be like to see a ghost and then to seeing angels. It became clear that LeeAnn was a member of a Christian tradition, which led to my asking, 'Do you ever talk to God?' LeeAnn discussed having an active prayer life and said her prayers were mostly about other people and about her CF. She said that she felt very connected to God, and that talking to God in prayer about CF helped her live with the disease. To better understand her relationship with God, I asked her, 'If God could come here, into your hospital room, and sit down in this chair like I am, what two questions would you ask God? Or, what two things would you like God to say to you?' LeeAnn's affect suggested both intrigue with the question and being temporarily at a loss for an answer. Since the visit had lasted approximately 30 minutes by this point, I suggested that she think about the question as 'homework' and asked if we might discuss it more at the next visit, to which she readily agreed.

The outcomes from this visit were a deepened relationship with LeeAnn, evidenced by her affect and her remaining engaged in the conversation and her willingness to continue the conversation. I began a narrative assessment process and understood that she had significant spiritual resources (belief in God, positive image of God, active prayer life), with relatively few spiritual needs identified at this point. At this institution, an ongoing chaplaincy relationship is an indicator for initiating a Patient Plan of Care (PPOC) goal against which progress would be documented at successive visits. The goal I documented at this time was, 'LeeAnn and/or her mother will verbalize impact of CF or current hospitalization on beliefs, values and relationships, and/or describe how she/they use spiritual or religious practices as a coping mechanism'.

Second encounter

Three days later, LeeAnn was alone in her room when I arrived. After I donned gown, mask and gloves to enter, LeeAnn immediately invited me to sit down and play a board game with her that was sitting on her bedside table. While setting up the game, she said, 'I thought of my question for God last night.' Her question was, 'What do you want me to do?' My follow-up question was, 'How do you think God would answer that? What do you think God wants you to do?' She shrugged and said, 'I don't' know,' and then, after thinking a moment, she said, 'Help others?' LeeAnn went on to tell a story of how she had helped a peer at school and how this made her feel good about what she'd done. She thought God would be pleased with her effort, too. I affirmed that God would be pleased by her helping others. After another turn or two at the game, the visit had to be terminated due to the arrival of a respiratory therapist to help LeeAnn do her airway-clearance treatment. We agreed I would return and to continue our conversation.

The most obvious outcome was LeeAnn's continued engagement with me, evidenced by her not only thinking about the question for God overnight, but initiating the topic for discussion during this visit. Her interest or curiosity had been piqued. Her response was noteworthy for having more to do with herself as a person than for having to do with CF. This question, 'If God could sit down in a chair with you, what two questions would you ask God?' (or the alternative, 'What two things would you like to hear God say to you?') has been helpful in creating a reflective conversation with adolescents. The question calls for some projection and the ability to think outside of one's self. Adolescents usually respond well to the question and to follow-up discussion that further explores their answers. The termination of this visit before the conversation could develop was unfortunate; however, LeeAnn's response suggested to me that she has an identity separate from the disease, which is a strength.

Third encounter

Ten days later, LeeAnn was using a laptop computer when I arrived, but she set it aside as I entered the room. She again invited me to sit down and play a game with her. Between turns, I asked about how she keeps from getting bored since she was expected to be in hospital another 7–10 days. She said that her grandparents were coming that night, that she likes to play games with nurses and staff, and that she likes to draw. I also inquired if she still felt like God was with her, or if she talked with God. After three rounds of the game (with other conversation between turns), I offered her two 'invitations' and said that she was free to decline either or both. The first was that 'We might talk to God and pray together', to which she nodded and said she'd like to do that. When asked what she wanted to pray about, she responded that she wanted to say 'Thank you' for a good pulmonary-function test that morning, since the score meant she was getting better, and for a safe journey for her grandmother, who would be driving a long way to spend the night with her. After the prayer, the second invitation was for LeeAnn to consider being part of this case study. I explained that the case study was about describing what chaplains actually do and what difference it seemed to make. I also promised her she would be able to read the manuscript and would be given a copy of the published version. She said she was interested, and that she was already part of one of the hospital's promotional videos, which she then showed me on her laptop.

The outcomes of this visit were a deepened pastoral relationship with me, evidenced by her setting the laptop aside when I entered the room, suggesting that she wanted to focus on our time together, and by her interest in praying. The fact that she had specific prayer topics, rather than a generic acceptance of prayer, suggested that she valued the opportunity. Her affect also went from flat to bright when I entered. The second outcome was her interest and assent for participation in the case study process. Here I followed the model previously used by Jay Risk whose case study was published only after the patient had read the manuscript and had an opportunity to comment on it (Risk 2013).

Fourth encounter

LeeAnn's grandfather was in the room when I arrived 3 days later. After some ice-breaking conversation, I commented on the drawings in her room that LeeAnn had done, and the markers and paper on the bedside table, and asked if she'd be interested in drawing together. After each of us had drawn a couple of pictures separately, I wondered aloud what it would be like to 'draw a picture of you when you are sick, and God'. LeeAnn's affect immediately brightened at the suggestion and she began to draw and, when she was finished, I asked her to explain it to me. LeeAnn had drawn a literal floor plan of her hospital room, with two angels keeping watch at the foot of her bed. She had colored the space on either side of the picture, above and below her bed, orange, which she described as 'heavenly light' which surrounded her. She described this light as the way in which she felt God was present with her all the time in the hospital. At this point, her grandfather entered the conversation and told a story of someone who had met an angel. LeeAnn said this positive, immanent imagery of the angels and continually being bathed in heavenly light were comforting images. I thanked her for drawing and discussing her work. Since this was the day prior to her expected discharge, I suggested that drawing might also be a way of feeling close to God, and a way of praying that she might continue at home. I asked if she wanted to pray together and, when she said yes, I offered a prayer using words from her description of her drawing (Figure 1.1), and we prayed in thanksgiving for God's presence with her and bathing her in heavenly light.

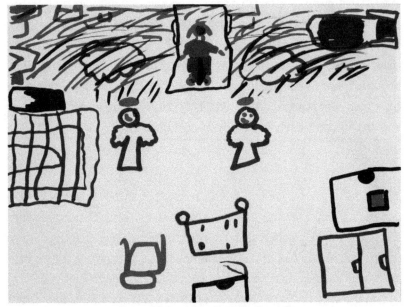

Figure 1.1 LeeAnn's drawing of herself

In her PPOC, I documented that her progress on her goal was 'adequate for discharge' since she had discussed and practiced 'spiritual/ religious practices as a coping mechanism' through prayer and drawing. The outcomes of this visit included a brightening of her affect with the suggestion of a drawing focusing on her, God and sickness. The drawing also allowed me to refine the spiritual assessment, having learned of her very positive and immanent sense of the Divine with her.

Fifth encounter

When I arrived on the floor the following day, LeeAnn had not yet been discharged. I entered her room and, after some initial conversation, pointed to the drawing from the previous day of God's presence with her when she was sick, and wondered what she thought about God and CF when she wasn't sick. She described God as 'telling the doctors to pick the right medicine' for her and said that she felt God continued to be present with her at home just as much as when she was in the hospital. This visit was terminated by the arrival of another professional who needed time with her prior to discharge. The outcome of this visit was an expression of her willingness to have me follow-up with her in 2 weeks at the post-hospitalization outpatient clinic appointment and the new information that she believed God acted for her healing by 'guiding the doctors'. She continued to speak with me about her faith and how it relates both to her disease and her life at home.

Sixth encounter

The sixth visit with LeeAnn and her mother took place approximately 2 weeks later in the waiting room of the outpatient CF clinic. This was my first opportunity to speak with LeeAnn's mother about the case study project. I described the case study to her mother, who gave her verbal permission for me to write it and submit it for publication. I explained that I would not be able to see them in the exam room that day since they were already scheduled for the maximum number of providers for that visit (an attempt by our CF team to limit outpatient appointments to less than 3 hours). The public nature of the waiting room somewhat limited our conversation, but it provided an opportunity to ask how school was going for LeeAnn and how she and God were doing. When I asked if they would like to pray about anything, they indicated that they would, and I offered a brief prayer of thanksgiving (based on how well LeeAnn's lung-function test had improved since discharge). The outcomes of this visit included brightened affect for both LeeAnn and her mother when I entered the waiting room, suggesting that they value our relationship;

creating connectedness with God through prayer and their changed affect and expressions of gratitude, interpreted as the prayer having had a positive impact on them; and obtaining the mother's permission for the case study to proceed.

Seventh encounter

About 5 months later, LeeAnn was admitted to the hospital with a bacterial infection in her lungs that significantly decreased her pulmonary functioning. The team expected she would be hospitalized for 2 weeks for intravenous antibiotic therapy. When I entered her room, she was using a laptop computer and indicated that this was how she was coping during the day. Board games were notably absent from the room on this occasion. She asked me if I could provide her with drawing materials and I said I would bring some on the next visit. The outcome of this visit included reestablishment of the chaplaincy relationship. My documentation in her PPOC was that LeeAnn 'will express through words or drawing…how she uses religious practices as a coping mechanism'.

Eighth encounter

The next day, I brought paper and markers and we both began to draw, with some conversation during the process. LeeAnn displayed considerable creativity in drawing and especially in storytelling about her drawings. Since she was expected to remain an inpatient for at least one more week, I asked if she would be interested in using drawing as a different way of praying and as a way to relax if she became anxious. She said she would, and the outcome of this visit was the agreement that I would introduce drawing as a different way to pray as an intervention at the next visit.

Ninth encounter

Two days later, I brought mandala outlines, including both preprinted designs[1] as well as simple circles for complete freedom in drawing. I explained that these were ways to combine into one activity two things she has said in the past were important to her: drawing and prayer. I further explained that this form of drawing allowed whatever she was feeling or thinking as most important to her at the time to come out in a form that could be seen and perhaps discussed. LeeAnn immediately took out the markers and began to draw.

Tenth encounter

The following day, I returned and, after some ice-breaking conversation, asked if she had finished the drawing she had started the previous day. She smiled and nodded and brought out several mandalas, which she had colored. I asked what the experience of drawing and praying that way had been like for her, and she replied that it had been 'fun' and that it 'takes a lot of time'. She also said that she would like to continue doing more of this. I reminded her that she could start new mandalas anytime by simply drawing a circle on a piece of paper. She described her favorite, which was colored like a sun, and associated it with 'home' and 'God'. The outcomes of this visit were that she showed she had accepted the invitation to try a new way of praying and demonstrated willingness to talk about the experience. My assessment reaffirmed that LeeAnn had a bright, immanent, positive image of God. I attempted to transition her towards independence in using mandalas by reminding her that she did not need to wait for me to bring preprinted copies for her.

At a subsequent outpatient clinic appointment, LeeAnn's pulmonologist and her mother decided on a new course of therapies. The frequency of her inpatient hospitalizations has decreased. One result is that I see her less frequently, since my primary clinical setting is the inpatient unit rather than the outpatient clinic. I do attempt to see her and her mother in the clinic to maintain our relationship, and I continue to see LeeAnn when she is admitted as an inpatient. We continue to talk about God while drawing or playing games. As she grows up, I expect there will be changes in how we talk about faith in the context of her disease.

Discussion

In this case study I present my work with LeeAnn because it typifies my approach in pediatric chronic illness chaplaincy. I deliberately avoided potential case studies that would have been unusual or extreme. I didn't consciously alter my approach with LeeAnn knowing I would be writing this case study. In my chaplaincy care I make use of what I see around me in a child's room to develop a relationship with them, as I did playing board games and drawing with LeeAnn. These clues also can be used to remind children of the sacred after they have returned home. I don't offer to pray in every encounter just to differentiate myself from professionals in other psychosocial disciplines.

Assessment

One of the strengths of Risk's (2013) chaplaincy case study is that he sets the case on a theoretical foundation, that of narrative theory. Risk's study is the first chaplain case to be set in a theoretical context. In a response I wrote about Risk's case (Grossoehme 2013), I cautioned about chaplains using a theory that did not arise from within chaplaincy and which was developed by another discipline; however, I am not aware of a stronger alternative theoretical foundation for chaplaincy care than narrative theory. In the interest of building on Risk's work, I have adopted narrative theory for the present case study, despite my desire for a more theoretical chaplaincy. In fact, it is the lack of such a theoretical foundation that motivates my desire to contribute to the case study literature. When a sufficient number of case studies are available for examination, perhaps it will be possible to develop a theory of chaplaincy that can serve the profession in the future.

In his presentation of narrative theory, Kleinman describes three archetypal narratives which people tell: chaos, restitution and quest (Kleinman 1988). Chaos narratives lurch from crisis to crisis, a cycle from which the narrator finds it difficult to break out, even when concrete forms of assistance are offered. Quest narratives have shifted from asking 'Why?' to 'What now?' They seek to learn from an event, however awful. The goal of a restitution narrative, of which LeeAnn's story is an example, is to return to life the way it was before and make things come out right.

It is necessary for chaplains and other clinicians to resist temptations to favor one narrative over the others; neither quest nor restitution narratives are inherently 'bad'. Furthermore, it would be a misuse of narrative theory to help the storyteller begin to tell a quest narrative, as if that is the end of narrative evolution and the goal of chaplaincy. Another narrative theorist, Arthur Frank, argues strongly for allowing the story to be told however the narrator needs to tell it, akin to the chaplaincy mantra of 'meeting the person where they are' (Frank 2009). I understood my role in these encounters as helping draw LeeAnn's story out, whatever story needed telling that day. Inquiries of 'How are you and God doing?' and 'Do you ever talk with God?' were means of helping her narrate her story. They were also a means, in my mind, of thinking about which narrative was being told, and then of deciding how to intervene.

Despite my familiarity with narrative theory, it did not occur to me until after my third or fourth encounter with LeeAnn that I might use narrative theory as an interpretive framework for my work with her. LeeAnn was not searching for answers; she was intrigued by the idea of asking God questions, but was not predisposed to seek any meaning or answers. Despite her multiple sinus surgeries and frequent outpatient CF clinic appointments, her description of her life and activities did not move from crisis to crisis; rather, her story about her life before our first encounter was quite similar to what she said she expected to do after each encounter, that is, return to her familiar activities and relationships.

I have had clinical encounters with other individuals, often shortly after traumatic injury or the trauma of a new diagnosis, in which the story of getting better and getting back to life the way it was seemed unrealistic. In my encounters with LeeAnn, however, restitution to her prehospital status seemed appropriate and that influenced my interventions.

Intervention

LeeAnn reasonably expected to return to much the same condition as before each hospitalization. Despite her frequent hospitalizations for acute issues, her lung function was relatively stable during this period. Her image of God was positive and she felt well connected to God and family. This suggested a focus on relationship building and maintenance for my care against the day when her situation might become more severe and make open discussion of existential questions more difficult without a prior relationship. My realization that her stories were consistent with a restitution narrative was accompanied by a choice of interventions which centered on relationship building and maintenance through facilitating her telling her story. It also suggested to me that interventions which explicitly integrated her 'secular' interests (drawing and playing) with the sacred dimension of her life would provide her with additional tools with which to tell her story or to cope with her disease as it progressed.

Establishing relationships with children is often done through play. As I have described elsewhere (Grossoehme 2013), play is a spiritual activity. When we are sick, our 'healthy self' goes into remission and our 'sick self' comes to the fore. Disease is a self-centered state: the focus is *my* pulmonary function, *my* breathing treatments, *my* body mass index. In play, we lose our self-centeredness and become who we truly are. Play also establishes community and, when engaged in by a chaplain in a *worshipping* community, is created because the relationship is grounded in the sacred. Play also offers an immediate, albeit temporary, end to the isolation of being alone in the hospital.

Playing with what is at hand (in this case, board games), and making intentional use of LeeAnn's obvious interest and skills in drawing, are physical expressions of 'meeting people where they are'. To the extent that drawing is an act of creativity, it is a godly activity. The introduction of mandalas was an attempt to provide an alternative, non-verbal means for LeeAnn to self-soothe and to pray in the hospital or at home and to link two parts of her life together.

People do not live in isolation, but are embedded in relationships. Nowhere is this clearer than in pediatrics, where a family-centered care approach means caring for the whole family, and not simply the person in the bed. LeeAnn's situation, however, was a challenge from that perspective. When she was an inpatient, she was normally alone during weekdays when I visited. Opportunities to be with both LeeAnn and her mother were limited to the outpatient clinic; however, due to the time constraints placed on non-physician members of the team during clinic, it was challenging for me to engage in a spiritual discussion with LeeAnn and her mother in approximately 8 minutes. Due to distance from home and his full-time work schedule, LeeAnn's father was not present in either the outpatient or inpatient settings when I was. He was normally present every evening during LeeAnn's inpatient stays. My focus, therefore, was on LeeAnn alone. This meant I was only able to hear one story rather than stories of all three members of this family, and to see how they were woven together.

One of the critical elements of narrative theory is that listening to a story impacts the listener. Engaging in self-reflection as I listened to LeeAnn's story was important (Kleinman 1988). I am the surviving older sibling of a brother who died from a congenital cardiac malformation for which there was then no repair. I grew up visiting his grave in the children's section of the cemetery where he is buried. I'm often told, 'Oh, that must be so hard to work at a children's hospital'. In contrast, part of what allows me to enter and listen to the stories of others is having heard a similar story from a very early age. Being told by others 'how hard' my ministry must be, or being told that I would 'get over' my brother's death has contributed to my willingness to allow others to tell whatever story they want to tell without challenge. Chaplaincy means accompanying them – listening, perhaps offering alternative explanations or commentary, or suggesting something that draws from my knowledge of where the person may be, emotionally or spiritually, at the moment. This is what lies behind my interventions and the way in which I offered them to LeeAnn.

Another aspect of my story stems from my undergraduate years, during which I studied astrophysics. Science and theology have been intertwined for me for several decades. I prefer a scientific explanation for illness over a theological one (e.g. CF is caused by a genetic mutation rather than by God, or God's will). I think it is a misuse of one story to use it to explain the other. So I am less interested in hearing stories about 'why or how we got here' than in 'now that we're here, what is this like?'.

Outcomes

Changes in her affect provided an easy means to monitor a key initial outcome, the development of a chaplaincy relationship with LeeAnn. While LeeAnn's narrative was largely filled with spiritual resources rather than needs, the development of a chaplaincy relationship out of which to function when the level of need increases was a primary goal of my care. Cystic fibrosis remains a life-shortening illness for most people with the disease, and the day may come when LeeAnn's narrative turns from one of restitution to chaos or quest. Listening to a restitution narrative now ideally creates a relationship out of which LeeAnn, or someone else, can feel safe enough to ask me questions about their quest journey, or to invite me into the chaos of their world turned upside down. A case can be made for prioritizing chaplains' care for persons experiencing spiritual struggle (Fitchett, Meyer and Burton 2000) who are likely telling a chaos narrative; however, in the case of chaplaincy with persons with chronic illness, it seems important to develop relationships by listening to their restitution narratives before, or between, chaos stories.

In our chaplaincy department, if a chaplain expects more than two encounters during an inpatient admission, the documentation guidelines call for the creation of a PPOC goal. In this case, the goal against which I measured progress (outcome) was typically: 'LeeAnn and/or her mother will verbalize impact of CF or current hospitalization on beliefs, values and relationships, and/or describe how she/they use spiritual or religious practices as a coping mechanism.' This was later modified to include the use of drawing instead of, or in addition to, verbal descriptions of coping. Throughout the period in which these encounters took place, the outcome of demonstrating the use of faith as a means of living with CF was also included. It should be noted, however, that this goal was created by me for LeeAnn. In healthcare, outcomes that are identified by the patient, or developed jointly with the patient, are becoming increasingly the outcomes of choice. In chaplaincy we have at least one model for spiritual outcomes developed jointly between the patient (or family members) and the chaplain (Lucas 2001), although this model has yet to be empirically tested for efficacy or effectiveness.

Case study issues

I received the invitation to submit a proposal for this case study shortly before LeeAnn was admitted for the first encounter described here. I queried the institutional review board at this hospital and I was informed that case studies do not constitute 'research', defined as the systematic research for generalization, and so did not require oversight from the hospital's institutional review board. I explained the case study project first to LeeAnn (during the third encounter described here) as an attempt to explore 'what chaplains actually do' and 'what difference it seemed to make'. I told her that the focus would be on me as the chaplain, that she could choose not to allow me to present the case study and that I would show her a copy of the manuscript before it was submitted. I told her that she could choose her own name for me to use as I wrote. LeeAnn smiled and appeared pleased with this request, and did not have any questions. I later approached her mother and explained the project again and obtained her consent to proceed. I mailed a copy of the initial draft of the manuscript to LeeAnn and her parents and invited them to let me know of any changes for clarity or accuracy. I invited LeeAnn to write a few sentences about these visits from her perspective. At a subsequent outpatient clinic appointment, her mother told me that she and her husband, and LeeAnn, had read the initial draft of the manuscript. They requested three clarifying changes: first, LeeAnn chose the pseudonym used in this case study to protect her identity; second, they requested clarifying language explaining that her father was not present in her room when I visited because he was at work and visited in the evenings; and third, that LeeAnn's cheerleading was part of their church rather than her school (as I had initially described it). I also told them that they would be provided with a copy of this book. After reading the initial manuscript, LeeAnn wrote, 'Thank you for telling my story. I really appreciate it! Thanks again, LeeAnn'.

My discussions with other professionals about this case occurred primarily in the weekly psychosocial inpatient rounds, where I reported that LeeAnn was working with me and that my focus was relationship building, providing community and strengthening existing spiritual resources. There were no issues that arose during our conversations which would have impacted her healthcare and which would have been reported to the other clinical team members.

Conclusion

A common saying in pediatrics is that 'they're not just little adults'. This statement is used to explain why the culture in pediatric healthcare is different than in adult health, and this should include a developmentally informed approach to chaplaincy. Such chaplaincy includes the integration of play and creativity, not for their own sakes but as means to build relationships or to mediate the sacred. This case study shows how play and creativity were used in this instance and records the evident outcomes. A limitation is that one of the most potentially important outcomes, LeeAnn's willingness to ask difficult questions when they arise in the future, is not knowable at the moment. More proximal outcomes, such as changes in affect and continued engagement with the chaplain, suggest that the interventions were at least efficacious (better than 'usual care', which would have been to have no chaplain visits). Future care for LeeAnn is likely to include strengthening the resources she already possesses and inviting her to develop her own voice by identifying aspects of her spiritual life that she may want to focus on in the future.

Endnote

1   These can be downloaded for free from the Internet (www.hellokids.com/r_262/coloring/mandalas-gallery-coloring-pages).

References

Ball, R., Southern, K.W., McCormack, P., Duff, A.J.A., Brownlee, K.G. and McNamara, P.S. (2013) 'Adherence to nebulised therapies in adolescents with cystic fibrosis is best on week-days during school term-time.' *Journal of Cystic Fibrosis 12*, 5, 440–444.

Bucks, R.S., Hawkins, K., Skinner, T.C., Horn, S., Seddon, P. and Horne, R. (2009) 'Adherence to treatment in adolescents with cystic fibrosis: The role of illness perceptions and treatment beliefs.' *Journal of Pediatric Psychology 34*, 8, 893–902.

Fitchett, G., Meyer, P.M. and Burton, L.A. (2000) 'Spiritual care in the hospital: Who requests it? Who needs it?' *Journal of Pastoral Care 54*, 2, 173–186.

Frank, A.W. (2009) 'The necessity and dangers of illness narratives, especially at the end of life.' In Y.O. Gunaratnam and D. Oliviere (eds) *Narrative and Stories in Health Care.* New York, NY: Oxford University Press, 161–175.

Grossoehme, D.H. (2013) 'Chaplaincy and narrative theory: A response to Risk's case study.' *Journal of Health Care Chaplaincy 19*, 3, 399–111.

Kleinman, A. (1988) *The Illness Narratives.* New York, NY: Basic Books.

Lucas, A.M. (2001) 'Introduction to *The Discipline* for pastoral caregiving.' *Journal of Health Care Chaplaincy 10*, 2, 1–34.

Modi, A.C., Lim, C.S., Yu, N., Geller, D., Wagner, M.H. and Quittner, A.L. (2006) 'A multi-method assessment of treatment adherence for children with cystic fibrosis.' *Journal of Cystic Fibrosis 5*, 3, 177–185.

Risk, J.L. (2013) 'Building a new life: A chaplain's theory based case study of chronic illness.' *Journal of Health Care Chaplaincy 19*, 3, 81–98.

Saiman, L., Siegel, J. and Cystic Fibrosis Foundation Consensus Conference on Infection Control Participants (2003) 'Infection control recommendations for patients with cystic fibrosis: Microbiology, important pathogens, and infection control practices to prevent patient-to-patient transmission.' *Infection Control and Hospital Epidemiology 24*, S5, S6–S52.

Stallings, V.A., Stark, L.J., Robinson, K.A., Feranchak, A.P. and Quinton, H. (2008) 'Evidence-based practice recommendations for nutrition-related management of children and adults with cystic fibrosis and pancreatic insufficiency: Results of a systematic review.' *Journal of the American Dietetic Association 108*, 5, 832–839.

US National Library of Medicine (2013) 'Cystic Fibrosis.' Available at www.nlm.nih.gov/medlineplus/ency/article/000107.htm, accessed on 4 July 2014.

Wilfond, B.S. and Taussig, L.M. (1999) 'Cystic fibrosis: General overview.' In L.M. Taussig and L.I. Landau (eds) *Pediatric Respiratory Medicine*. St. Louis, MO: Mosby, 982–990.

Chapter 2

'I can tell *you* this, but not everyone understands'

– Erica, mother of a 2-year-old girl with cancer

Alice A. Hildebrand

Introduction

This case study explores a spiritual care relationship that developed over a year and a half with Erica, the young mother of Macy, a 2-year-old girl with a very serious cancer. My visits occurred weekly when Macy was an inpatient. Initially, Macy's admissions were approximately a month long; as her treatment progressed, they lasted about a week. There was one lengthy period when Macy was not in the hospital and I had no contact with Erica or Macy for several months. My visits were usually 30–45 minutes long.

The hospital where I work, Maine Medical Center (MMC), is a 637-bed level-one trauma center in Portland, Maine, which includes the Barbara Bush Children's Hospital (BBCH), the only full-service children's hospital in Maine. Maine is a very rural state, with a depressed economy. It is the third least religious state in the USA (Rogers 2013).

The Spiritual Care Department at MMC includes a director, who is a board certified chaplain and a clinical pastoral education (CPE) supervisor, and two board certified interfaith chaplains. From September to June we are joined by interfaith chaplain residents for an extended (part-time) unit of CPE. The staff chaplains and the CPE students cover patients in assigned clinical areas regardless of the patient's stated religious preference. The department also has Roman Catholic priests and a Roman Catholic Sister who are employed by the Diocese of Portland, as well as a communal Jewish chaplain supported by the local Jewish community. The Roman Catholic and Jewish chaplains cover the entire hospital but provide services based on religious preference. Prior to the time of this case study, the patients and families of BBCH had been served only on an 'on call' basis, since BBCH has very few patients who list any sort of religious preference.

I am a 60-year-old white woman who has lived in rural Maine since 1974. I became a United Church of Christ minister in 2001 after having been a recorded minister in the Society of Friends (Quaker) for 8 years. I am board certified by the Association of Professional Chaplains. I currently serve as the chaplain to the Women's and Children's Service Line of MMC, which includes BBCH and the prenatal, labor and delivery, and mother/baby care/newborn areas.

My care of Erica and Macy occurred several years ago during a pilot project I undertook with the support of my director, Rev Catherine F. Garlid, and Dr John Bancroft, Chair of Pediatrics. I wanted to see what difference it would make for patients, family and staff care to receive routine support rather than 'crisis only' support. This project included a partnership with the outpatient oncology site, the Maine Children's Cancer Program (MCCP). The pediatric oncology patients of BBCH are followed by physicians and social workers from MCCP, both as outpatients and inpatients. These patients receive intensive social work support in both settings, but before this project they did not have much access to a chaplain (unless by specific request), due to the way the provision of spiritual care at MMC was structured. The project created a model in which the chaplain worked closely with the social workers for the care of pediatric oncology patients.

McCurdy and Fitchett (2011) have recommended that chaplains request consent from the subjects of their case studies. Consistent with this I made several unsuccessful efforts to contact Erica by phone to describe my plans for this case study and to request her consent. Next, I discussed this situation with key MMC staff including the Chief of Pediatrics, the Director of Clinical Ethics and the Director of the Spiritual Care Department. All of those people felt that proceeding with the case study without Erica's permission was acceptable as long as details about the patient and family were disguised. I also discussed my plans for the case study with a social worker who was still working with the family. She read an early draft of the case study and felt that the family's privacy was sufficiently protected. The names used in the case study are pseudonyms.

Because this is a case study about my work as the chaplain on the case as much as it is about Erica, I have organized the presentation of the case around the different roles that I played.

Case study
The chaplain as representative of the familiar

Erica, a woman in her early thirties, asked for a chaplain's support when she came through the emergency department with her daughter Macy on Macy's first admission. The on-call chaplain responded to this request and then referred Erica to me for follow-up. When I first met them, Macy had just had major surgery and was in much pain. Erica was attentive and creative in her caregiving, managing to distract, soothe and anticipate her child's needs. She was dressed in cargo pants and a flannel shirt, and proudly described herself as a 'redneck', which is a message about where she locates herself in the present societal matrix of the USA: 'I am a down-to-earth, working person'. But Erica had also been employed as an assistant in medical settings and had more education than the 'redneck' label implies. She was clearly knowledgeable about the procedures her child was undergoing. She was insightful and articulate about her child's needs and her own needs. She was appropriately assertive on behalf of her child and not intimidated by the medical environment, holding Macy in her arms throughout procedures. She partnered effectively with the medical team and was well liked by the staff.

Very early in our relationship, Erica told me that it was her faith in Jesus that was making it possible for her to cope with Macy's illness. She also told me some of her life story, which included living on her own at a very young age. She had an older daughter whom she had raised as a single parent, until she married her present husband, and several other children. However, most of our conversation (unusually so in my experience of the patient population of BBCH) was about religious topics, including matters of biblical interpretation and theological concepts such as the meaning of the Trinity. Several years before our encounter, Erica had had a powerful and direct experience in which 'God spoke to [her]'. She felt that God had carried her through earlier trauma and would carry her now. She told me that she didn't bother talking about her religious faith with the other providers taking care of Macy, as she didn't feel anyone but the chaplain would understand what she was saying. She kept an angel doll with 'Jesus loves me' embroidered on its chest hanging from Macy's IV pole, and told me that that was a way of 'witnessing' (to her faith) when they were in the corridors or the playroom.

The chaplain as mother/guide when the familiar is lost

This verbatim segment, from a visit 2 months into our relationship, represents the beginning of a turning point. Our initial encounters had always included praying together, at Erica's request, but this visit was the first time when it felt as though we weren't quite praying as equals, but that either she trusted me enough to let me see her vulnerability or her need was so great that she couldn't hide it. During this and in subsequent visits, I assumed a 'motherly'/pastoral role with Erica (who is young enough to actually be my child).

Chaplain: Hey, Erica, good to see you! Hi, Macy! Look at that great hat you have!

Erica: That's her indoor hat, now that she has no hair.

Chaplain: How are things going?

Erica: Well, this time she's nauseous, we've been throwing up all night, every 3 hours, but we haven't worn any yet, have we, Macy? She doesn't like throwing up, and she wants to just lie there, but I don't want her to aspirate so I make her sit up and get it out. But the good news is that we're going home today.

Chaplain: When was the last time you were home?

Erica: I stole a little time yesterday and went to see my other kids. I had the most amazing experience, I went past my house a little way – I'd never done that before – and I found a church. I go into churches all the time, I'm always looking, but I mean this time, I found one.

Chaplain: That's great!

Erica: I was driving and I saw this sign and then it was a really, really long drive and I was thinking it must be a wrong turn, and I was thinking that I should go home and see my kids, but it was like a very small, still voice was telling me to just keep going, so I did, and suddenly, in the middle of all these woods, there was an enormous church!

Chaplain: (*nodding*)

Erica: And the service was half over, but I went in anyway, because I do that, I don't ever feel embarrassed anymore when I go into a church since I had my experience where God spoke to me that time I told you about. And I got there and everyone's head was bowed, and they were having prayers, and the first thing I heard was 'Prayers for [person's name], having chemo…' and then for five more people having chemo, and I knew I'd found the right place.

Chaplain: You felt like you were where you needed to be.

Erica: Yes, it was so amazing, because I really had almost not kept going, but the voice kept telling me to go, and then I found it. It was just so amazing that I almost didn't go and then when I did, I found what God wanted me to see. Like, what if I hadn't gone down my road just a little farther like I did that day so that I saw the sign?

Chaplain: It's like the story of Moses and the burning bush. He was just out tending his father-in-law's sheep, doing his job, and he noticed a bush on fire, but not burned up, and he turned aside from what he was doing, and *then* God spoke to him. God didn't yell, 'Moses! Come over here!' But when Moses stopped to look, then God spoke to him.

Erica: (*Nodding, smiling, playing with her hair.*) Yes, exactly, that's cool. This lady came up to me afterwards, when I was leaving, and tried to get me to stay, and I told her, 'I'll be back, but I have to go now, my kids need me, but I'll be back, God brought me here.' I don't mind telling church people that anymore – and she was like, 'Oh'…but friendly. (*Addressing me.*) I know you understand, I can tell *you* this, but not everyone understands. My friends really don't understand, some of them are like, 'Oh you're just acting'; some of them are like, 'That's too weird' and some of them just don't know what to say. But since that day when God spoke to me, I've never, ever doubted. The day that God spoke to me I went into work and my supervisor took one look at me and he just knew and he let me go off and read the Bible all day.

During this conversation, Macy had been playing with extra medical supplies and toys on her bed, and watching cartoons. She began to say 'Mommy' while we spoke, and every time she did I smiled at her, and she smiled back. So it became a game that she and I were playing, while Mom talked on, and that seemed to content her.

Chaplain: So, you were saying that a lot of people close to you can't really relate to this part of you. How is it for you with Eddie [her husband]?

Erica: Well, he can't really get what happened for me, but he gets it that I really had the experience. He's the only person who knows me now that knew me then, and he knows how much I've changed. Like, I was never somebody that said, 'There's no plan, it's all random', but I didn't know if there was a God or gods or just some big universal plan, and now I really, really know. But I don't know why God would speak to *me*…so I don't really share this with Eddie.

Macy was becoming more insistent and Erica began to talk to her in between sentences, still telling me about how God was living in her and making her strong and able to do this, alternating with small talk with Macy about her cache of thermometer covers, syringe caps and so forth. Macy spotted a box of Frosted Flakes next to me on the bench and wanted it, and she and I played back and forth, passing the cereal to each other and growling like Tony the Tiger (the figure on the box).

Chaplain: Well, Erica, I should be going, too. Would you like it if we prayed?

Erica: Always.

Erica was standing near me holding Macy and there wasn't an easy way to hold their hands as I usually did, so I put my arms loosely around them both.

Chaplain: Beloved God, we thank you for your presence here with us. We thank you that you are always with us, everywhere, and that you are holding Erica and Macy in your hand. We ask a special blessing on Erica and Macy, and Eddie, and all their family.

At this point I became aware that Erica was crying, and she cried through the rest of the prayer. I drew the prayer out so that she could really cry. She never got loud or vigorous and Macy never acted alarmed. It all felt very peaceful. I gradually held them fairly closely to me, rubbing Erica's back while I prayed. By the time the prayer ended, Macy, who has no eyebrows anymore, was playing with mine and touching my face lightly.

Erica: (*Putting Macy back on the bed and wiping her eyes.*) Well, we'll be leaving really soon, but we'll be back for the next cycle.

Chaplain: I'll come see you again. (*Fist bump with Macy.*) Take care of yourself.

Erica: I will!

Another day's visit included the following exchange, in which I used our discussion of a potentially dry topic, which translation of the Bible is 'right', to try to reach into Erica's life experience.

Erica: I don't like all these Bible translations, you know? Only the King James, I don't know why they have all these other ones, because that is the one that is right. And the modern ones, they change it all, because they have a different context, they mess with it…like the New International Version…it doesn't even say that Mary was a virgin, and that's kind of the whole point, right? It just says that she was a young girl!

Chaplain: Well, that is the original language, in the Hebrew, where the image comes from. All these translations, like you said, they all have a context, and so it is important to know what the contexts are so you can really get the story…like the original manuscripts don't have any punctuation or paragraphs or even spaces between words, and so for me, what's so special about the story of Mary is that even though she was an unwed teenaged girl, she had the vision and the courage to say, 'My soul magnifies God!' – to really stand up and say what she felt God doing in her and for her.

Erica: Yeah, that is so cool! I never thought of it that way. So she was like a single parent might be, kind of, at least in the beginning.

The chaplain as team member

As I got to know Erica, it became apparent that some of her reluctance to share her faith with others in BBCH came (as she shared in the verbatim above) from prior experiences of rejection from people with whom she had shared her beliefs. Despite her outgoing and apparently confident demeanor, and despite her eloquent statements about her strong relationship with God, my assessment was that she was generally very sensitive to the possibility of being judged as unacceptable and/or inferior in some way, and of her faith being dismissed by others. Her bravado about being a 'redneck' was one indication; her silence with the social workers about her faith another; and still another came early on when she compared me with the first chaplain whom she had met in the emergency department, saying that chaplain was dressed 'too fancy' (i.e. in a skirt and blazer, with nylons, dress shoes and a necklace) and it made her uncomfortable, whereas my simpler outfit of black jeans, turtleneck and fleece was 'friendlier'.

I also wondered about the possible reasons Erica might have had for not wanting to share some of the details of her life with me. Years of working with people in recovery from drug and alcoholism issues, their own or another's, have made me very aware of certain clues in people's accounts of their lives, what is unmentioned as well as what is described. I had an intuition that part of what Erica was not telling me involved substance abuse, past or present. Since I am a person in long-term recovery, I thought carefully about what I might disclose of my own past in order to open a door for Erica to share more with me.

An opportunity came one day when one of the social workers called me to say that Erica was looking for help for one of her older children and was hoping to find a Christian counselor. When I next saw Erica, I told her that I didn't know of anyone who would be described as a Christian counselor and that my own bias would be to find a counselor with a good reputation for working with young teens, rather than looking by religious preference. This led to a thoughtful conversation about her concerns for this child and some of the dynamics in her family, including her husband's past difficulty with substance abuse and its lingering effects on their family.

Erica's absence from home, as she accompanied Macy through the maze of treatment, meant that her other children were not under Erica's close supervision and care, and this was creating a crisis. Fortunately, Macy was handling treatment quite well; Erica said one day, 'Right now Macy is actually the healthiest one in our family.'

I reflected the anger towards her husband that I heard from her and Erica said a bit more. Her husband arrived and, as he entered the room, Erica picked up a Nerf gun lying on Macy's table and shot him in the chest with its foam darts, four times in quick succession. He appeared intimidated and made an awkward joke of it. She told him that since he was there with Macy she and I would leave and go outside so she could smoke. Once in the smoking area, she picked up where we had left off. I mentioned Al-Anon as a possible resource and as something that had been very helpful to me. She was mildly interested but didn't ask any questions. She finished her cigarette and we went back inside.

The chaplain as mentor and spiritual friend

That was the beginning of a new pattern for our visits. We would go out so Erica could have a smoke, and in that setting, she explored issues from her past and the challenges her family faced in addition to Macy's illness. After several times of not having much privacy in the designated smoking area, we moved to a quiet street corner and would sit on the curb and talk. Sitting side by side, with her taking great care not to let her smoke drift into my face and always taking any trace of her cigarette away with her, we shared a deeper kind of conversation than we had previously. We never had very long conversations, and she often began her story sort of in the middle, but my goal was to listen intently to what she needed to say, not to analyze it, so if I missed some of the sequence or logic, it was OK with me. Our posture (next to one another, both looking out into the street and only sideways at each other), our location (curbside, on the same level) and my lack of comment on her smoking were part of the creation of a very safe and accepting space.

In that space, I shared some of my own past with Erica, in the manner familiar to me from years of 12-step-program work, in which a person who has been in recovery for a while speaks to a person who may be beginning to wonder about recovery issues in their own life, not by telling the other person what to do but by describing what they themselves have done. In these conversations, I was very clear internally about two different kinds of role authority upon which I drew: one based in the norms and patterns of 12-step work, the other based in the norms and patterns of chaplaincy as I practice it. In either role, the goal of any self-disclosure made by me is to benefit the other person.

One day, as Macy was nearing the end of her rounds of treatment and was shortly to be discharged to go to another hospital for another procedure, Erica shared with me questions she had about her own use of substances. I told her explicitly what I had done to end my own use and when we parted the next day, for what would likely be several months, I gave her some Alcoholics Anonymous meeting lists for her area. But I did not give her my home phone number nor did I offer to take her to a meeting, both things I might have done were we only meeting in a 12-step-program context. The context of our meeting was Macy's admissions to MMC, in which Erica's goals were the treatment of her child's illness. This meant that my work with Erica was limited to supporting her as she supported her child; it was not appropriate to focus in much detail on addressing any issues that Erica herself had. (If I had felt that Erica was in imminent danger at any time, this stance would have changed and I would have worked hard to get medical care for her via the emergency department of MMC.)

Several months went by during which I had no contact with Erica and Macy. When Macy's procedures at the other hospital were concluded, and the last phase of chemotherapy began, our relationship resumed. Following both my own style as a recovering person and my sense of appropriate boundaries as a chaplain, I did not ask Erica whether she had gone to any 12-step meetings. In the 12-step context, my belief is that the person who is considering recovery has the right to move at their own pace and to elect whether or not to attend meetings. In the chaplaincy context, my belief is that the recipient of spiritual care is in charge of what they reveal to the chaplain and when they reveal it. In either context, if Erica had not chosen to take the route of 12-step meetings, I might have damaged or cut off our relationship were I to have led with that question. My goal was as before – to meet her where she was and see what use I could be to her, which would have included actual confrontation of substance abuse issues if I believed that might be useful.

Macy was now receiving her chemotherapy in the intensive care unit so that side effects of this final round of treatment could be carefully managed. Much of the time she was uncomfortable and unhappy, and Erica did not leave her. But when she was asleep or comfortable enough to play with a nurse, Erica and I would go outside to our curb. Our conversations were quickly on the same level as before. The effort she and her husband were putting into their own relationship, as well as the extra support being given to their other children, meant that despite Macy being in a risky part of treatment, Erica was much calmer. It was during one of these conversations that Erica acknowledged that she had not previously allowed herself to feel hopeful about the outcome of Macy's cancer. As the rounds of chemo were completed, Erica began to talk about what a return to normal life would look like for her family, the need for a larger house, her hopes that her father could move and be closer to them and the start of school for one of her other children. Our visits began and ended with hugs.

As treatment drew to a close, I explored several times with Erica what the support system of her 'normal' life would look like: the new church home, the chance to be part of extended family activities and a possible change of community if a larger house was purchased. Life would not be completely normal in that Macy would continue to have periodic clinic visits and at least one of the social workers would remain involved with the family. But the intense, inpatient world would end. I was consciously and carefully inviting her to consider the issue of whether leaving that world of cancer treatment and its support system would feel like a loss. Nothing that she stated or implied led me to feel that it would be.

Our relationship ended in a quiet way as Erica and Macy were leaving the hospital for the last time. She and her husband gave me a large, framed photograph of an ocean scene, full of light and motion. It was a fitting symbol of the time we had spent together. We said our goodbyes, had our hugs and they left.

Discussion

Assessment

In developmental terms, human beings move in infancy from the intense dependency upon their primary caregiver for nourishment and nurture to an ability to nourish and nurture themselves. Winnicott (1984) described the process of attachment and separation as a lifelong challenge, which is enhanced by the discovery and use of 'transitional objects/transitional phenomena'. Transitional objects, such as the 'blankie', teddy bear or other soft toy, are familiar symbols which provide comfort, love and connection as the toddler begins to separate from the primary caregiver. As teenagers and adults we find stimulation and comfort in ideas, the arts, religion, creative work – 'transitional phenomena' – which helps us to create and enjoy our unique identities, to soothe and distract ourselves from pain or fear. Issues of attachment and separation surface over and over again throughout our lives and can be particularly troublesome during times of stress, such as illness.

Illness forces us into a confrontation with the meaning of attachment and separation against the backdrop of the mystery of life, as well as the attachments of human love and identity against the separation of death. Gregory Fricchione has identified ways in which a physician can assist patients as these needs are triggered:

> The physician becomes in effect a transitional object, a symbolic parental presence of protection and guidance. As a result, the doctor is imbued with the power to transport the vulnerable individual faced with the specter of separation and loss of attachment to a safe

place, ideally within some higher, more mature level of attachment.
(Fricchione 2011, p.5)

Chaplains, too, can function as transitional objects for patients and
families in the crisis of illness, whether a family is religious or not. If
a family is religious, then the chaplain may also serve as a symbolic
presence and reminder of the protection and guidance of God.

Throughout my initial meetings with Erica, she never expressed
any fear for her daughter. As noted above, it was not until treatment
was nearly over and our relationship had deepened that Erica told me
that for the first time she had hope that Macy would survive her cancer.
In early visits, Erica's almost ecstatic expression of faith dominated our
interactions. Her primary need seemed to be to reiterate her absolute
faith in God's sovereignty and loving care. My analysis was that it was
comforting to her to be able to affirm with me as a chaplain her world
view that God was in control, and therefore, whatever happened would
be the right thing. The fact that the medical team was able to quickly
resolve Macy's pain post-surgery and that Macy responded well to
chemotherapy treatment also helped Erica affirm the 'rightness' of what
was happening, despite the fact of the cancer.

Initially, Erica coped by armoring herself with her faith as a way of
managing her feelings. During the beginning phase of our relationship,
she frequently requested grace over meals and prayers for herself and
her daughter. Since Erica was often standing holding Macy on her hip
while she visited with me, as described in the verbatim above, once we
ended up with my arm around them as we prayed, and Erica cried quietly
throughout the prayer. After that, she would more or less launch herself
into my arms when we prayed, and would cry quietly throughout. She
needed 'mothering' from the chaplain, a symbolic reminder of God, and
the context of prayer allowed her to ask for and receive it. However, it
was clear to me, first from the chart notes and team meetings with the
social workers, and then from Erica herself, that unmet spiritual needs
were buried underneath her familiar comfortable religious language
and imagery. Consequently, I worked to help her articulate those needs

during our interactions, at the pace and depth of her own choosing. What emerged throughout our year and a half of visits were significant issues of loss: deep loneliness in her past; substance abuse; and much pain over the present situation of her children, who were coping with issues of their own, and over Macy's very serious cancer. But her lack of expressed anger at God and of any doubt about God's agency in her life as a force for good seemed genuine. She was able to hold onto her faith in God's wisdom and care even as she described these life events. As we established a trusting relationship she allowed me to represent God's love. I, as the chaplain, was the person who helped her to interpret her life – in the present, with its challenges and grief; in the past, with its significant triumph over adversity – in the religious language and traditions that were so important to her and in a way that, using the language and expertise of their various disciplines, none of the other caregivers could.

Interventions

Working in partnership with the social workers who were supporting Erica and her family (at one point, there were three of them involved: one for Erica, one for Eddie and one for them as a couple) made it possible for me to simply listen to Erica much of the time, as opposed to also thinking about psychosocial diagnosis and treatment goals. There were times when, upon readmission, she would begin talking to me about a present situation without giving me many details of the weeks in between our visits. All I needed to do was listen and not distract myself with curiosity about any of the gaps in the storyline. What was healing and helpful to her was to have me receive the information, not to analyze it.

As our relationship developed, I used my instincts about what might be part of her inner world to share some of my own history as a way of inviting her to greater openness. I also believed that if she did indeed have issues of addiction that needed to be addressed, she would need to deal directly with those, and that the 12-step model, with meetings free of charge, easy to access and emphasizing spiritual growth, would be a very positive place to begin that work.

Interestingly, as our relationship deepened, she stopped asking me to pray with her, although we continued to talk a lot about faith on the experiential level. The locus of holiness moved out of religion and into life, perhaps in a way similar to our relocation from Macy's room to the streets, where Erica could smoke and talk freely. In my interactions with Erica on the curbside, it was always clear to me, and seemed clear to Erica, that I was the chaplain and not a 'recovery peer', despite my self-disclosure and the many points of contact between my past and hers.

Outcomes

At the time of Macy's final discharge, many of the difficulties in Erica's home situation had been resolved. I attribute this to the intra-psychic and spiritual work that Erica and Eddie did with the social workers and with me. Despite Erica's willingness to disclose her own substance abuse history and her questions about it in seeming response to my self-disclosure as a recovering person, she never shared with me anything about attending 12-step meetings of any kind, nor did she return to the topic. I cannot evaluate whether she did indeed need to directly address her substance use, but I believe that my self-disclosure was appropriate and helpful, as the depth and breadth of our conversations greatly increased subsequent to that conversation. During this time period Erica also found a worshipping community that felt comfortable and welcoming to her. While we never explored in detail her stated dissatisfaction with the many churches she visited, as we established a trusting relationship, which included very open discussions about religious and spiritual matters, her search for a church home ended satisfactorily.

Conclusion

As my relationship with Erica progressed, my goal was to get religion out of the way so that spiritual care could begin. While I never doubted that Erica's sense of connection to a loving, powerful and wise God was vivid and real, and helpful to her, I felt that the issues and feelings she was sharing with the social workers needed to be brought into her dialogue with me. I believed that articulating to me her fears for her children, her anger at her husband, as well as her yearning to connect deeply with him, and her feelings of shame and inadequacy about her past would strengthen and enrich her connection to God. Sharing those things in the context of a spiritual care relationship, as well as within the counseling model employed by social workers, added different dimensions of nurture to a very challenging situation.

My work with Erica illustrates the model of spiritual care which informs my work as a chaplain. It is my goal to be aware of, and attentive to, feelings and needs that may be buried beneath a person's initial self-presentation as a person of faith. I seek to convey to the patients, families and staff with whom I work that I am available to move beyond religious conversation to this deeper layer. This can occur with patients who I see only once as well as with patients with whom I have multiple visits, whether the patient is distressed by past experiences brought to light by the crisis of a hospital admission or by feelings newly created by the admission itself. Because the relationship I had with Erica was a long one, we were able to move slowly past the starting place of her request for religious support. Initially, she wanted prayer and a person with whom it would feel safe to share a religious interpretation of what was happening to her daughter and who could represent God's care and commitment in an intentional way. As our relationship progressed, other dimensions were added.

It is my role as a chaplain to make it absolutely clear that if someone wants to go to a deeper level, I will go with them. I will not keep us on the surface for a need of my own. In order to make that tacit commitment to another, I have to be very sure that I can follow through with it. So I believe that the most important part of the work I will ever do is *inner work*, plumbing my own fears and chaos so that I will not pull away from the fears and chaos of others.

Erica was living with significant stress and distress, and she made superb use of all the resources offered to her. Her statement to me early on, 'I know you understand, I can tell *you* this, but not everyone understands', illustrated her assumptions about the type of person with whom she could discuss matters of faith. Several times she articulated this rationale for her decision not to talk about faith with the social workers and other members of the healthcare team. What was never articulated was why she initially chose not to disclose life and family stressors to me. My theory was that doing so would have caused her to feel shame, and so I used careful self-disclosure as a means of normalizing some of her life experience. Overall, my assessment was that she initially called on a chaplain to help her remain grounded in the faith that had carried her through bad times before. Then, as our relationship deepened, she allowed me to serve as a 'transitional object' and 'mother' her through some very bad times. Finally, after I had shared some of my own life with her, and as Macy's treatment drew to a successful close and the challenges the family was facing were somewhat resolved, Erica engaged with me as a mentor and spiritual friend.

References

Fricchione, G.L. (2011) *Compassion and Healing in Medicine and Society: On the Nature and Use of Attachment Solutions to Separation Challenges*. Baltimore, MD: The Johns Hopkins University Press.

McCurdy, D.B. and Fitchett, G. (2011) 'Ethical issues in case study publication: "Making our case(s)" ethically.' *Journal of Health Care Chaplaincy 17*, 1–2, 55–74.

Rogers, A. (2013) 'Where Are the Most Religious States in America in 2013?' Time NewsFeed. Available at newsfeed.time.com/2013/02/13/where-are-the-most-religious-states-in-america-in-2013, accessed on 4 July 2014.

Winnicott, D.W. (1984) 'Transitional objects and transitional phenomena.' In D.W. Winnicott (ed) *Through Pediatrics to Psychoanalysis: Collected Papers*. London: Karnac, 229–242. (Original work published 1951.)

Chapter 3
'Why did God do this to me?'
– Angela, a 17-year-old girl with spinal injury

Katherine M. Piderman

Introduction

The subject of this case study is Angela, a blond, blue-eyed, petite 17-year-old girl. An average student in her last year of high school, she had been involved in athletics but hadn't excelled; she had some friends, but was considered by many an 'outsider' who didn't fit in well. Angela's parents had been divorced for several years and she lived with her mom and her older brother and younger sister. Angela and her mom were often at odds and they had had an argument the morning of her car accident. Angela said that she 'tolerated' her brother and sister but didn't feel close to either of them. She had little contact with her father, who lived in another state, and she described him as 'a loser'. The relative she was most fond of was her grandmother, who was at the time in a nursing home recovering from a fractured hip.

Angela was admitted to hospital after she lost control of her car on an icy highway. The car, with her belted inside, went over an embankment and rolled three times. Angela was conscious when the emergency personnel arrived, but she was unable to move. She was extricated from her car and airlifted to the nearest tertiary care hospital. Scans determined that Angela's spinal cord was severed at a high cervical level and she was paralyzed from the neck down. When Angela was medically stable, she was transferred from the intensive care unit to the physical rehabilitation unit for therapy, where her projected length of stay was 3–4 months.

Angela wore a brace that stabilized her neck and spine, but the medical team did not expect Angela's paralysis to improve in any way. She required assistance with all personal care, including bathing, grooming, dressing, and bowel and bladder needs. She was admitted to the rehabilitation unit with the expectation that she would participate in six sessions of rehabilitation each day. During these therapies, she was to be given guidance and skills to prepare her to make the transition to life outside the hospital. Angela's mother had been present for only a few of these sessions and it was not clear who would have primary responsibility for Angela's care after discharge or where she would live.

Angela had visitors most evenings. Her mother and a few of her mother's friends came to see her. Her brother and sister each came twice. Her pastor had come once and her father was expected later in her hospitalization. Friends sent Angela cards, but none visited following her transition to rehab. Angela's grandmother called her frequently.

I am a staff chaplain with 40 years of ministerial experience (20 years as a pastoral minister and 20 years as a chaplain). I work at the Mayo Clinic in Rochester, Minnesota, a large academic medical center in the midwestern United States. I am endorsed for ministry as a chaplain by the Roman Catholic diocese in which I live, and I am board certified by the National Association of Catholic Chaplains.

When I met Angela, I had been working on our rehabilitation unit for 7 years as part of an interdisciplinary team focused on providing the best holistic care for patients with spinal cord injuries, brain injuries and other conditions requiring inpatient rehabilitation. My role on this team was to conduct spiritual assessments and facilitate and/or provide spiritual care. I initiated visits and received referrals from patients, families and the team when spiritual matters relevant to the course of treatment arose. I also communicated insights and interventions to the rest of the team, and helped to develop the plan of care for each patient.

Preparation and publication of this case study was approved by the institution for which I work. While the case study is based on my ministry with a real patient, to protect her confidentiality, and in accord with the policies of our institution, I have used pseudonyms throughout the case. In addition, some demographic information and other details about the case have been omitted or altered. The case study was not reviewed by our institutional review board because a case report involving one individual is not considered research.

My interaction with Angela took place over 5 years ago. It was so rich and meaningful for me that I made detailed notes and wrote a verbatim about my experience with her. Since that time, I have had several occasions to use this material in teaching clinical pastoral education students, staff chaplains, medical students and psychiatric residents about various aspects of a chaplain's ministry. This case demonstrates the unique role a chaplain can serve with patients, especially those with religious concerns. It also shows the way the existing literature on spirituality can inform clinical practice and guide interactions with patients.

Case study

At the time of the meeting described below, I had seen Angela four times. My initial goals in these visits were to build rapport with Angela, to get to know her and to understand the role of spirituality and religion in her life, especially at this time. My approach to this kind of very basic spiritual assessment is framed by the FICA Spiritual Assessment Tool (Puchalski and Romer 2000). The FICA helps chaplains and other professionals gather basic information about the spiritual and religious background of patients by using questions similar to these: (1) Do you have spiritual or religious beliefs that help you cope during this time? (F: faith); (2) What importance do your beliefs have for you at this time? (I: importance); (3) Are you a member of a spiritual or religious community? What is that like for you? (C: community); and (4) Are there any particular spiritual or religious activities that are important to your well-being while you are in the hospital? (A: activities). I weave such questions into conversations with patients, like Angela, to elicit and note information that describes their spiritual and religious needs and expectations during their hospitalization.

To deepen my understanding of patients, I also use my own 4C Spiritual Assessment Tool which leads to a discussion of how people feel *centered* or anchored, *called* or motivated, *connected* to relationships beyond themselves and *contribute* to the good of the world and/or the good of others, in small or grand ways. I ask how these aspects of their personhood are helpful to them, put them in struggle and have been affected by their injuries and/or hospitalization. With Angela these discussions were only very preliminary, but I expected to engage in these issues more as my relationship with her developed.

I learned that Angela was a member of a small evangelical Protestant church in her hometown. She went to services and Sunday school when she was young but was no longer an active church attender. She still considered herself as a Christian, but, prior to her car accident, she rarely thought about God or prayed, even though her grandmother nudged her to do so. Following the accident, Angela had been trying to get closer to God, and stated that she prayed several times each day and that she appreciated the prayers of others. She had a Bible her grandmother had given her at her bedside. Because of her limitations, Angela could not pick it up or even hold it herself, but she did ask people to read it to her occasionally. The pastor from Angela's church had visited her, but she didn't feel very connected to him. She was open to my visits and had asked me to come to see her every day that I could. She stated that she enjoyed talking with me about her newly burgeoning faith and about how God was working in her life.

Initially, Angela seemed to be coping adequately with her injury, but as often is the case with any profound loss, she seemed distant from its permanence. At my first meeting with her, Angela told me that her mother had said to her, 'God never gives you more than you can take' and 'If you pray hard enough, God will give you a miracle'. Angela had adopted these beliefs and they fashioned her hope. She said, 'I'll do what they want me to do in rehab, but I know I won't have to stay long. I'll be better soon.' Then, she believed, she would have an important witness story to tell. At Angela's request, I prayed with her for the miracle everyone wanted, but I also asked that God give Angela what she needed in the meantime.

The visit outlined below took place at the end of the second week of Angela's rehabilitation. It was initiated in response to a referral from the psychologist working with her. Though Angela had been compliant with therapy during the first 10 days, for the last few days she had refused therapy, including grooming and bowel care, and had eaten and drunk very little. She had been told that especially the latter choice had potentially life-threatening consequences, but she said she just wanted to be left alone. Her willingness to engage with the psychologist, known for his sensitivity and compassion, was nil. Finally, she dismissed him, saying several times, 'You don't understand.'

I prepared for my visit with Angela with the expectation that it would be difficult, and indeed it was. One of the advantages of a well-functioning interdisciplinary team is that there is usually at least one member who can be effective with even the most challenging patients. My hope was that my previous time with Angela would help her to trust me. I prayed that I would have the grace, strength and insight to engage with her in a way that would be helpful.

On the previous occasions I had visited her, Angela had greeted me with a smile and seemed glad to see me. But this day, she barely acknowledged my greeting. I expressed my concern that she seemed 'down'. She nodded but didn't say a word. I pulled up a chair beside her and we sat quietly together. Within a few minutes, tears began to flow from Angela's eyes.

Angela: I'm so mad! And even though I can't move, I have pain and tingling all the time. It's not fair! It hurts a lot!

Chaplain: I'm so sorry, Angela. Your situation is very difficult. Tell me more about what it's like for you.

Angela: I feel so trapped! I hate my life! There's nothing I can do! (*sobbing*)

Chaplain: What is the hardest part for you, Angela?

Angela: Everything! Just everything! And I can't even wipe my tears.

Chaplain: Would you like me to wipe your tears?

Angela: No! There's nothing you can do. There's nothing anybody can do. Why isn't God answering me? This is more than I can take! I hate being like this!

Chaplain: I hate this for you, too, Angela. Your situation is so difficult and I can understand why it feels unfair. You've lost so much.

Angela: I've lost everything! Absolutely everything. (*She continues to sob. Her neck is the only part of her body she can move and she tenses it in positions as far back and forth and up and down as her brace will allow. I sit quietly beside her.*)

I am mindful of Eric Cassell's view of suffering as a threat or experience of destruction or disintegration of the self (Cassell 1991). Angela's words speak of the assault of her condition on herself as a person. It was much more than a physical injury. Compounding her distress was her loss of a 'spiritual center' that could anchor her. She had grown weary of the wait for a miracle and felt overwhelmed by the challenges of each day and her concerns about the future. Though she focused on not being able to wipe her own tears, it seemed that this was symbolic of the many intrusions on her young body that defied privacy and threatened personhood. For Angela, my offer to wipe her tears represented my desire to be helpful to her in a tangible way, an 'easy way', and she may have interpreted it as missing or minimizing her real suffering.

Cassell states that suffering continues until the threat passes or is integrated into the self in some transformative way. In Angela's case, unless the prayed-for miracle occurred, it seemed that the latter transformative process would be necessary for her suffering to be relieved. The goals of my ministry with her became more focused with this realization.

The powerful barrage of Angela's emotion was a bit daunting to me. My hope was to find a way to guide Angela to integrate her suffering so that it would eventually lead to the healing and restoration of her sense of self. I realized that this would be a long process, but I also knew that her stay in rehab would give us time. I remember reaching deep inside to center myself in my belief that God is with us always, and perhaps especially in our deepest darkness. I wanted to be present with Angela and faithful to her in her darkness, but also to help her find what centered her.

> *Chaplain:* Angela, you have told me that your mother believes that God is helping you with this and is expecting God to give you a miracle. Do these beliefs help you at all today?

> *Angela:* No! Absolutely not! (*Then, she pauses and reflects.*) Well, not really…I just don't know. I just don't know. I'm so confused. I know what my mother thinks and her friends, but when they pray over me – well, it's just weird. I feel nothing, and it's scary. They think prayer is magic, hocus pocus or something like that. Well, they're wrong. Their prayers aren't working and neither are mine. Then they tell me that I have to be strong and that God won't give me more than I can take. I wish they'd just leave me alone.

> *Chaplain:* It's so hard when things don't work out the way we expect, especially when we're counting on them. We will certainly support you if you want to restrict their visits in any way.

> *Angela:* I know they mean well, but when God doesn't answer our prayers I feel that I must have done something terribly wrong. I know I haven't been the best person, and I did have that fight with my mother the day I crashed my car, but I haven't been bad enough to deserve this. And I don't know why God would ever think I'm strong enough for this. I'm not! I'm not! I'm not! (*She begins to sob again.*)

Chaplain: You're thinking about really important things, Angela. It seems like you're trying very hard to understand why the accident happened, why you're so badly injured, and what God is up to in all of this.

Angela: You're right! I want to understand. They say that there must be a reason. I feel so hurt by God. Betrayed. (*sobbing*) Why did God do this to me? My life was already hard enough. What more does God want from me? I've always tried to be good. Why did this accident happen? They tell me that it says in the Bible that God won't give you more than you can take, but this is too much! How am I supposed to live like this?

Angela sobbed while I sat with her silently. In part, my silence was intended to honor Angela's suffering and to give it the space and respect it deserved, but I was also considering how to proceed. Angela's anguish was apparent on many levels. Physically, she had the many challenges that paralysis brings and she also had pain. Emotionally, she was enraged at her plight, especially her helplessness. She felt profound despair as she looked ahead to the future. Spiritually, she felt devastated by God's silence and apparent absence. This was compounded by her sense that God was responsible for her situation. Her initial means of spiritual coping (i.e. borrowing her mother's beliefs) was no longer working for her and she had nothing to put in its place. She felt bereft and hopeless.

Angela had trusted me with her raw and uncensored grief. At this point at least, she had not painted me with the same brush that she had painted her mother and her mother's friends. I had chosen to acknowledge her trust with statements of acceptance and understanding and by remaining physically present beside her. I know that this was a powerful means of ministry and may have been enough for her, at least for that day. At the same time, I wondered if Angela's questioning could have had an element of questing within it and some desire to grapple with the mystery of suffering. Angela's sobs subsided, and I decided to find out, ready to retreat to a more supportive stance if she resisted.

Chaplain: You have so much anger and so many questions. In situations like this, your answers have to come from within you, not from someone else, not your mom or her friends or me or anyone else.

Angela: It's horrible. Everything is horrible.

Chaplain: It's so dark for you, Angela. You thought you could count on God to get you through and even change things, but now it seems as if that isn't going to happen, and worse, that God is the cause.

Angela: That's it exactly.

Chaplain: Suffering is so hard to understand. We always have more questions than answers in the midst of it. Usually any answers we have aren't enough to take away the pain, but still somehow it seems important to voice the questions and the feelings we have about them. I'm so glad that you're doing that with me. Would you like to take a question or two and work with them and see if we can find some light, some hope, as we do?

Angela's sobs had stopped, and she looked at me and nodded.

Chaplain: Where would you like to start?

Angela: I don't know. I don't know. There's so much I don't understand. I think the worst thing is that people are telling me that this is all part of God's plan. I don't get it. I don't deserve it. Why did God do this to me?

Angela was again bringing up her belief that God was responsible for her accident and injuries. I was aware that this perspective clashed with mine, which was based on Romans 8:28, 'We know that in all things God works for the good of those who love Him, who have been called according to His purpose.' My experience has taught me that 'the good' is often not apparent during times of suffering, but with time it may be revealed. I bristle to think of some who may have used their beliefs about 'God's plan' to suppress any protests Angela may have made about her existential plight. I also know that I am not comfortable with the belief that God orchestrates every event in our lives. I believe that it is more likely that God is with us to guide us in and through them. I wanted to offer this perspective to Angela for her to consider, but I knew it would be wrong to impose it on her or to criticize her present beliefs. My intention was to tread softly and slowly, and see what she was open to.

Chaplain: That seems like a good question to be asking. Do you think God caused the accident?

Angela: Well, yes. I mean, no...not really, I guess. It was icy and I just, I just went off the road on the corner. It was my fault. I was mad at my mom and not paying attention. I'm so sorry. (*She began to cry again, but with what seemed like sadness rather than anger.*)

Chaplain: I know that you're trying to make sense out of things and that it is very confusing for you. This is the first time I've heard you talk about your responsibility for the accident. It must be a heavy burden for you. Driving on ice is difficult for all of us, especially if we're mad and distracted. I'm sure if you could rewind the time before the accident or even at home you would, so would I, but we can't and we're stuck with the consequences of what has happened. Eventually, we're better off if we let go of our guilt burden. Does that make sense?

Angela: Yes, I guess so, but why did God break my spine?

Chaplain: Oh, my...do you think God reached into your spine and did the breaking?

Angela was silent and I worried that my words, based on my beliefs, had been too confronting or had pushed her too hard, but then she spoke.

Angela: Well, no, but why is it God's will? And why does God think I can take it?

My sense was that Angela was using our conversation to look at huge questions that had haunted her in the past weeks and perhaps in other experiences of adversity, such as her parents' divorce. She was struggling to make sense of what she believed, separately from what she had been told, and was being told, by adults in her life. Her crisis had hurled her out of secure reliance on these perspectives and onto the cusp of what James Fowler calls 'Individuative-Reflective Faith' (Fowler 1981, pp. 174–183). I wasn't sure if this was the time to give her more information to consider, but I was aware that her anger and sobbing had subsided, and that she seemed engaged. My goals were to respect her, be attentive to her and offer compassion, but also to challenge her in a way that might open new doors to God's grace. I decided to offer her my perspective.

> *Chaplain:* People believe different things about the meaning of God's will. I believe that God's will for us is always related to what is truly good for us, but that in the middle of a painful situation, especially one as painful as yours, it's hard to find the good. With time, though, we might see it. Does that make sense?

> *Angela:* No, not really. (*Anger returning.*) Why is God doing this to me?

> *Chaplain:* I don't know if this is true for you, but sometimes we ask questions when we're too mad to really seek an answer.

Angela was quiet and turned away from me. I wondered if, in my desire to give her a hand out of the darkness of her suffering, I had gotten ahead of her. She hadn't budged from her position that God was directly responsible for her accident. She did not seem ready to look at other options. Then she turned back to face me and spoke.

> *Angela:* Yeah, you're right. I don't really care what the answer is. I still hate it. I guess I just want to be mad.

> *Chaplain:* Is that OK with you and what you believe?

> *Angela:* Well, I don't know. Is it OK to be mad at God?

> *Chaplain:* I can't speak for you or for God, but I know that in Scripture there are several people who were mad at God, and Jesus certainly spoke of His feeling of abandonment on the cross. There are also several psalms that direct anger and disappointment to God. Anger

is often part of a process and part of a faith journey. It isn't necessarily the end of the story.

> *Angela:* Where does it say, 'God doesn't give you more than you can handle?'

I was aware that Angela had raised this theme several times previously. I was also aware of my negative reaction to it. That was perhaps why I hadn't explored it with her. It seemed to me to be more like a saying on a greeting card than a theological statement. In my experience, it can inhibit or deter helpful reflection on the meaning of events and suffering. To my knowledge, the closest Scripture reference to God not giving us more than we can take is 1 Corinthians 10:13:

> None of the trials which have come upon you is more than a human being can stand. You can trust that God will not let you be put to the test beyond your strength, but with any trial will also provide a way out by enabling you to put up with it.

I didn't want to make the mistake of turning my time with Angela into a catechetical session, but I wondered if it would be helpful to discuss this Scripture with her. I decided to give it a try.

> *Chaplain:* It doesn't exactly say that in Scripture, but would you like me to read the passage most closely connected with those words.
>
> *Angela:* Yes.
>
> *Chaplain:* (I read 1 Corinthians 10:13.) What do you hear in that?
>
> *Angela:* Well…that others have been through things like this before. Like Josh. It always helps when he visits. (*Josh is another rehab patient who is about Angela's age and has similar injuries.*)
>
> *Chaplain:* I'm glad you two have met and have a good connection.

I was now aware that Angela's relationship with Josh may be a catalyst as she moved in the direction of making her faith her own.

> *Chaplain:* Do you hear anything else in the passage I read?

Angela: Yes. That God will give me a way out or help me deal with it. I'm praying for a miracle and lots of other people are, too. But my mom says that I just don't have enough faith or I'd be healed already. (*sobbing*)

Chaplain: What do you think?

Angela: I don't know. Josh says that it's just not time yet, and we have to pray for patience and strength.

Chaplain: Does that help?

Angela: Yes. A bit. At least it helps that Josh tells me what he believes and that he prays for me.

Angela looked up at me and said, 'Would you help me blow my nose?'

Chaplain: I'd be glad to. Tell me what works best for you.

Angela explained, and I did as she directed, realizing how much I take the ability to blow my own nose for granted, and how humbling this must be for Angela. Then Angela asked me to help her wash her face and I did that, too. Angela sighed and looked relatively at peace.

Angela: That feels better, so much better. Thank you.

My sense was that what felt better was more than physical. I had a decision to make about closing the session or inviting Angela to talk more about her experience. I voiced both options to Angela.

Chaplain: I'm glad you're feeling better, Angela, and I thank you for your trust today. I've learned a lot about you and your courage to tackle difficult and scary questions. Have you had enough for today or would you like to talk more?

Angela: I think that's enough. I've got a lot to think about. Would you come to see me tomorrow?

Chaplain: I'll be glad to. May I pray with you before I go?

Angela: Yes, please.

Chaplain: Gracious God, in this time of suffering, please bless Angela with your love. Bring her healing and bring her peace. Give her, dear God, all that she needs to move forward and through her trials. May she always know that you are right beside her, as her friend and as her guide. Bless those who care for Angela. Give them compassionate hearts and skillful hands. Bless the other patients on this unit, especially Josh. In Jesus' name, we pray.

Angela: Thank you.

Chaplain: See you tomorrow.

Subsequent visits

When I saw Angela the next day, she was sitting up in her wheelchair, well groomed and smiling. She had resumed all therapies and was eating and drinking and accepting personal care. Though it was obvious that Angela's despair had lifted, I chose not to comment on the changes in her that were so evident. Instead, I asked her how she was. She responded, 'Pretty good. Better than yesterday.' Probing a little more, I asked, 'What do you think happened?' She looked down and seemed to withdraw a bit, but then looked up and said, 'I just understand better.'

As is often the case on a rehabilitation unit, our visit was curtailed by the arrival of a therapist for a scheduled appointment. When I returned to see Angela later in the day, she talked more about her 'understanding'. She said that not everything about her accident or her injuries made sense to her, but that she found herself singing the song 'On Eagle's Wings' inside herself. She knew that somehow God was helping her, but she also knew that she had to do her part. It seemed like calm had come to Angela after the storm. I was relieved for her, but I also expected that there would be much more struggle ahead.

I continued to visit Angela several times each week. My goal was always to be a sign of God's incarnational love, accepting Angela each day as she presented herself and offering her support, respect and compassion. In addition, I was attentive to opportunities to help Angela find God in the midst of her situation. My hope was to encourage Angela to explore and establish a relationship with God that would center and sustain her when she left the hospital.

Angela remained open to, and appreciative of, my visits with her. She openly expressed her feelings of confusion and frustration with 'God's plan' for her but did not seem as burdened or confined. I invited her to explore the images in 'On Eagle's Wings' and she seemed to find a consolation and direction in them. Visits with her mother often provoked distress in Angela, but she stated that she felt more confident that it was alright for her to believe differently than her mother. She also said that she'd always 'sing a little louder' after her mother had left.

One day, when I went to Angela's room, Josh was with her. Their therapies were done for the day and they were talking together with the cheerful animation common in adolescents. It was delightful to observe. I saw not two disabled teenagers, but two teenagers, who happened to have disabilities, enjoying each other as persons. I hesitated to interrupt, but I knew that Josh was close to his discharge date and I wanted to arrange a time to see him before he left. I also wondered if there might be a way to talk with both young people together, even briefly, that would be more beneficial than conversation with each individually. I knocked on the door and Angela invited me to join them.

After some preliminary pleasantries, I commented on their apparent enjoyment of each other. They agreed that they had developed an important friendship and said that they intended to keep in touch after Josh's discharge. Josh commented on his plans to finish high school and begin college. He wanted to find a way to fulfill his dream of being involved in veterinary medicine. Angela's discharge would not be for several weeks and much remained undecided, but I asked her if she had any thoughts about what she hoped to do when she left the hospital. She looked away from us and said, 'I don't know.' Then she began to cry. Josh spoke first and said, 'Angela, it won't be easy, but God will help you find your way.' His statement led to their discussion of the raw, Job-like feelings that Angela had struggled with on that earlier dark day. Josh had faced these feelings as well and his insights as a peer slowly, but surely, led

Angela to greater understanding, acceptance and peace. I entered into the conversation only when I thought it would be helpful to clarify something or support one of them. It seemed evident that their engagement was very fruitful without my direct involvement.

Angela's discharge was complicated because of her physical condition, her social situation and because she was a minor. I advocated for an arrangement that would provide the most certainty that Angela would be safe, physically, psychologically, socially and spiritually. Angela's mother did not indicate a willingness or an ability to oversee her care, and arrangements were made for Angela to go to a long-term rehabilitation center near her hometown. This was difficult for Angela to accept. I provided support and encouragement as she adjusted to what had been decided, and did what I could to help her prepare for what was ahead.

As the time came to say goodbye to Angela, I was aware of my sadness. I expected that the future would be difficult for her. I had often wished that my role extended to the outpatient area so I could maintain some supportive contact with patients. I recognized, though, that this boundary was important. I knew that it helped me guard against the temptation to over-function and take unrealistic responsibility for trying to make things work out well for patients. It reminded me that there were other patients to serve, and it also led me to lean on my faith that God would provide what Angela needed. Most of all, it helped me to be mindful of my gratitude for the holy intersection of persons that my ministry as a chaplain provides.

Discussion

During the visit described in the verbatim, Angela expressed rage, sadness and confusion at the circumstances in which she found herself. She was just beginning to understand her severe limitations and the need she had for others to care for her in both broad and very personal ways. Her resistance to this was evident in her refusal of therapy and personal care. To allow such things would imply that Angela had acknowledged and accepted her need for assistance. Her refusal to let me wipe her tears at the outset echoed this resistance, but it also revealed a deeper suffering (i.e. Angela's desperation for some sense of control, even if it was just in finding an explanation for what had happened to her). Her request for help at the end of the visit indicated that she was in a more secure and accepting place. Her re-engagement in the rehab process indicated that she had sufficient self-esteem to view her caregivers as an extension of herself, rather than an intrusion on her agency. This bode well for her post-discharge quality of life (Augutis and Anderson 2012; van Leeuwen *et al.* 2012).

In some ways, Angela's experience paralleled that of Job. Initially, she expected God to be faithful and cure her, but as time passed, she became discouraged. She felt abandoned by God and misunderstood by her mother and her mother's friends. Though she didn't beg to die as Job did, she wondered how she would go on living. She did not have the confidence in her relationship with God that Job did, and did not engage with God directly; however, she expressed her anger and despair to me, a chaplain and God's representative. Her peace at the end of the visit suggested that she had an experience of God that was much more subtle and gentle than that of Job. Perhaps it was more like Elijah's experience on the mountain when he discovered God in 'a tiny whispering sound' (I Kings 19:12–13) or more like an 'Emmanuel experience', (Matthew 1:23) the sense of God with her. It did not bring Angela a cure or restore her to life as she has known it, but it did restore at least an increment of her sense of self and her spiritual well-being. During her hospitalization, Angela continued to raise questions related to theodicy and continued to be open to discussion and growth in her perceptions. These were also hopeful signs (Kim *et al.* 2000; Johnstone and Yoon 2009).

Angela's accident and injuries thrust her into the age-appropriate developmental stage of ego identity (Erikson 1950). The intense feelings she experienced, inherent in trying to understand and accept her uniqueness and her separateness from others, were compounded by the existential anxiety her present situation had provoked. Without a clear sense of herself, Angela encountered anger and anxiety related to managing each day, and even more so the future. I saw reasons to be hopeful in her continued willingness to engage with me; in her openness to Josh's mentorship; and in her ability to reflect on her experiences, acknowledge inconsistencies in her thinking and move on to new perspectives (Augutis and Anderson 2012; Kennedy *et al.* 2012). Though her distress was profound at times, she had not even passively indicated a wish to be dead, but rather her question cited in the verbatim, 'How am I supposed to live like this?' seemed to imply that she expected and planned to live. She had also begun to consider how she had been called by God, and what opportunities she had ahead for personal fulfillment and to contribute to the good of others and the world. Though she did not leave the hospital with complete clarity about these issues, I felt that we had at least cleared a path so that she could continue the process of discernment.

My main concern for Angela was related to research findings that demonstrated a drop in existential well-being in persons with spinal cord injuries 6 months after their discharge from a rehabilitation unit (Piderman *et al.* 2011). To do well, Angela would need to continue to use active coping, including dialoging with others (Augutis and Anderson 2012). I hadn't been successful in helping Angela reconnect with her pastor. She simply didn't like him. The relationships between Angela, her mother, siblings and social network were tenuous at best and did not seem to supply her with the emotional support that she needed. I was concerned and wondered who would be available to help her deal with the issues of meaning and purpose that would inevitably be a part of her journey. Angela and Josh were committed to staying in touch and their relationship seemed mutually helpful. Perhaps there would also be a way that Angela's grandmother, whom Angela trusted and who had her own experience of disability, could have regular contact with Angela, even if it was only by phone. Her caregivers may also have new roles to play in providing support for her.

As I reflected on my experience with Angela, both shortly afterward and as I prepared this case study, I was struck by several things. First, I was keenly aware that my previous professional and personal experiences helped me minister to her. I had worked closely with adolescents during 20 years of parish ministry and was familiar with developmental challenges and the turmoil they bring. Years of working with people with various medical challenges, including spinal cord injuries, and being part of the team on the rehab unit, gave me some comfort and confidence in working with Angela. I had reflected frequently on the spiritual questions related to theodicy, both with patients and within myself, and Scripture was a gift that had guided me to more peace and acceptance of suffering's inherent mystery. Second, it was clear to me that despite my background, I did not have answers for Angela. While remaining present to her, in the midst of my conversations with her, I needed to 'step back' periodically to think about what was happening in her and in me, and to choose my response. This was not easy, especially when Angela was most distressed and when my beliefs were different from hers. There were times when I felt that my responses to her missed the mark, but because of our mutual commitment to the process and God's grace, we were able to go on. Third, I was aware that my encounters with Angela blessed me deeply. She trusted me with her suffering and helped me understand her plight in a way that was rooted in spiritual meaning. She invited me to be with her, but she also was open to exploring possibilities beyond her perspective. Because of my experiences with Angela, I was more equipped to minister to others on the rehab unit and understand my role on the rehab team. Several years afterward, when I was in a car accident similar to Angela's, memories of her helped me to cope with my own injuries, which fortunately were much less severe than hers.

Conclusion

Chaplains have the opportunity to minister to people during very difficult times. In this case study, I demonstrated my commitment to Angela by remaining present, open, faithful and steady while she railed against her situation and tried to find a path through it. I entered Angela's darkness with her while keeping my eyes on the light of hope. In this way, I put into action my belief that God is with us in the deepest of darkness and journeyed with Angela as she claimed this belief as her own. I reflected on my experience of being with Angela while I was engaged with her. I explored my own beliefs as well as various theories and research in an effort to try to understand Angela's plight and to find guidance for my ministry. My goal was to be helpful and compassionate while also inviting Angela to explore the mystery and possibilities before her. Along with the rest of the rehab team, I offered her the shelter and support of 'eagle's wings' during her initial terror and despair, but I also trusted that it was important to nudge her forward to find and use 'wings' of her own.

References

Augutis, M. and Anderson, C.J. (2012) 'Coping strategies recalled by young adults who sustained a spinal cord injury during adolescence.' *Spinal Cord 50*, 3, 213–219.

Cassell, E.J. (1991) *The Nature of Suffering and the Goals of Medicine*. New York, NY: Oxford University Press.

Erikson, E.H. (1950) *Childhood and Society*. New York, NY: W.W. Norton.

Fowler, J.W. (1981) *The Stages of Faith Development: The Psychology of Human Development and the Quest for Meaning*. San Francisco, CA: Harper Row.

Johnstone, B. and Yoon, D.P. (2009) 'Relationships between the brief multidimensional measure for religiousness/spirituality and health outcomes for a heterogeneous rehabilitation population.' *Rehabilitation Psychology 54*, 4, 422–431.

Kennedy, P., Lude, P., Elfstrom, M.L. and Smithson, E. (2012) 'Appraisals, coping and adjustment pre and post SCI rehabilitation: A 2-year follow-up study.' *Spinal Cord 50*, 2, 112–118.

Kim, J., Heinemann, A.W., Bode, R.K., Sliwa, J. and King, R.B. (2000) 'Spirituality, quality of life, and functional recovery after medical rehabilitation.' *Rehabilitation Psychology 45*, 4, 365–385.

Piderman, K.M., Mueller, P.S., Therneau, T.M., Stevens, S.R., Hanson, A.C. and Reeves, R.K. (2011) 'A pilot study of spirituality and inpatient rehabilitation outcomes in persons with spinal cord dysfunction and severe neurologic illness.' *Journal of Pastoral Care and Counseling 65*, 4(2), 1–13.

Puchalski, C. and Romer, A. (2000) 'Taking a spiritual history allows clinicians to understand patients more fully.' *Journal of Palliative Medicine* 3, 1, 129–137.

van Leeuwen, C.M.C., Kraaijeveld, S., Linderman, E. and Post, M.W.M. (2012) 'Associations between psychological factors and quality of life ratings in persons with spinal cord injury: A systematic review.' *Spinal Cord 50*, 3, 174–187.

Chapter 4
Critical Response to Pediatric Case Studies
A Chaplain's Perspective

Alister W. Bull

These pediatric case studies open a window into healthcare chaplaincy practice that demonstrates the impact such encounters can have when chaplains bring a perspective to the multidisciplinary team that is distinct. In relation to chaplains interested in the way others conduct spiritual and religious care, they provide insight into both what is common and what is different in each of their practice. For instance, the use of a theoretical framework is common to all, but how it is applied reveals some differences in approach.

The following observations address how reflective practice can develop insight and trust for all the chaplains; however, there are two further aspects of this practice that explore more specifically how the presence of pastoral power and a religious focus can be handled differently by each chaplain.

Features in common

Each of the chaplains used a theoretical framework to reflect upon their visits. This enabled them to engage reflectively on their practice and, to some extent, *in* their practice – so much so that each used their particular framework to develop subsequent encounters and thereby deepen their appreciation of the pastoral relationship. From their study of chaplaincy practice, O'Connor *et al.* (2005) suggest that frameworks are often formulated early in the chaplain's training, and that thereafter a chaplain will adapt and formulate their own approach to assess a patient. They identified that chaplains, in their practice, made an assessment of a patient using either an adopted or intuitive theoretical framework. Chaplains might use a reflective practice as an interpretive framework to understand the component parts of a pastoral encounter. This then allows the chaplain to deconstruct their practice in order to give meaning to how they in turn can engage with a patient. I wondered, in the light of this study, at what point these three chaplains adopted such a framework, and whether it was their only one. What seemed most obvious was the method of reflection. Less explicit, and slower to emerge, was their latent philosophy of chaplaincy. Grossoehme states, 'Chaplaincy means accompanying them – listening, perhaps offering alternative explanations or commentary, or suggesting something that draws from my knowledge of where the person may be, emotionally or spiritually, at the moment.' Like Grossoehme, the other chaplains seemed to have a settled viewpoint and these cases did not change their practice but rather confirmed that their approach to care was appropriate. If this is the case, it would be interesting to know how and at what stage they developed their intentional philosophy of care and the ways in which their theoretical framework has informed their thinking about their role as a chaplain, whether to parent, carer or patient.

What remains consistent across these pediatric case studies is that all of them consider not just the patient but the whole family in relation to the care. The case studies illustrate that, while seeking to be all-encompassing, the chaplain may not have fully grasped the family picture. This did not necessarily detract from the care given, but a fuller family background may help a chaplain engage with each member of the family in a more considered way.

I wondered about the incident in Hildebrand's case, where she complies with Erica's request to leave the father with Macy. Is spiritual care just to one member of the family or for the whole family? I would suggest that the offer be made and the choice be given; however, some chaplains may view this as compromising the pastoral relationship if the relationships within a family are strained. A possible way to resolve this question may be to have another member of the chaplaincy team involved. A discussion with the multidisciplinary team may also offer a wider picture and reveal how to appropriately offer care.

What is significant in each of the cases is how the chaplain documented the way they felt they had contributed to the well-being, recovery and peace of the patient and family. Grossoehme described what he sensed was involved in the process of repeat visits, beginning with 'relationship building and maintenance', and later refers to what he achieved as a 'deepened pastoral relationship'. In his opinion, the prospect of a long-term relationship was a key intentional principle in offering care; yet what seems more apparent was his intention to discover ways for the 12-year-old to cope using religious ritual as a resource in what is a rather restricted context.

Grossoehme's observations of the young person's 'affect' became a repeated assessment of his impact of care. This was illustrated by how he hoped, on the basis of his pastoral care, that 'she would feel free to ask religious/existential questions'. This shaped his practice, but it left me wondering how transparent the process had been between what he calls 'a narrative assessment process' and that of the more formal way as a Patient Plan of Care. The other cases had a similar dynamic: in both Grossoehme's case and that of Piderman there was an official hospital assessment and then a more personal assessment used by the chaplain. Each chaplain describes their assessments, but all I can deduce from this is that they have different functions. In my own studies (Bull 2012), it was apparent that healthcare chaplaincy has not reached the point where there is an agreed collective approach to assessment, and that there is a varied practice in documentation between the chaplain and the multidisciplinary team. The result of this disparity is illustrated in all three of these cases: in each there is an internalized assessment that is strongly relational and subjective and documentation that is outcome based.

What is evident in each of the cases is the different ways in which the chaplains strove to gain the trust of the one they visited. Grossoehme did this by spending time with the young person in a joint activity. Hildebrand describes the progression of her encounter on the levels of disclosure made by the parent. In my view, Hildebrand's approach reflects more the counseling culture of her social work colleagues than her own approach to care. The patient's sharing with the chaplain information about her past had a strong therapeutic impact on her and gave her the strength to cope because the chaplain helped explain the patient's understanding of her difficult circumstances. This is more an observation than a criticism, but the difficulty with this is that it may weaken the distinctive contribution that healthcare chaplaincy can bring.

Pastoral power

Another aspect to these case studies is the place of power and control – what some may refer to as the chaplain's professional authority to shape the direction of care, and what Michel Foucault calls 'pastoral power' (Foucault 1982). Within the chaplain-patient relationship, pastoral power is exercised through the use of religious language and concepts, and can either empower or disempower.

In the first two cases the place of power lies with the chaplain, while in the third case it appears to be quite different. The irony of this is that in Piderman's case, the patient is so completely powerless that it made the chaplain acutely aware of her own power. Hildebrand helpfully states, 'my belief is that the recipient of spiritual care is in charge of what they reveal to the chaplain and when they reveal it'. Despite that comment, I felt that all three cases raised questions of power, as the documenting of the patient or parent indicated what little control they had over the care they received. The use of the reflective framework helped the chaplain more than it did the patient. The choice of language used by the chaplains to describe their role (e.g. 'homework', 'mothering', 'this goal was created by me') further indicates where the balance of power lies.

The projected intention of the chaplain's caring role places the power more with the professional carer than with the person visited. The possession of prior information also increases a place of power as Grossoehme was obviously party to the religious profile of the patient. Even Grossoehme's affirming the patient's view of God or guiding these visits towards prayer could indicate subconscious power plays on the part of the chaplain.

This is not to suggest that there was any abuse of power, and it may be argued that the chaplain's power could be used to empower the patient. Hildebrand's prayer and physical contact certainly illustrated the tension of this possibility, and yet I could identify more closely with Piderman's points of physical contact. It has left me undecided. Physical contact can be such an important means of communicating care, yet its non-verbal dimension can be misunderstood on both sides.

In relation to Hildebrand's case study, I am concerned about her analogy of the chaplain as a transitional object. I would argue the chaplain should facilitate a transitional space to avoid dependence and rather create a place of interdependence; otherwise, paternalism in a pediatric setting can leave a chaplain exposed in a spiritual care role that is hazardous. I understand that a chaplain is part of that space, but if they lose their awareness of their liminal role, then they become emotionally involved, and that compromises their capacity to care and be ready to care for the next patient or visitor.

Religious focus

What is present in all three cases is the religious focus, either directed by the chaplain or in the chaplain's response to the patient or the carer. The emphasis each chaplain placed on 'God' illustrates how the interpretative framework can be blurred or focused, and how important it is to understand what is meant when referring to a deity and the relationship inferred by a patient making reference to a faith figure. The introduction of religious belief and biblical narrative allowed the chaplains to narrate and deconstruct (in the Derridean sense of the word) the life of the patient or parent through questions and reflection. For example, both the way Grossoehme seeks to apply his religious framework to address appropriate religious pastoral care and the way Hildebrand regards Erica's religious language as unhelpful in that it disguised buried and 'unmet spiritual needs', are deconstructive.

Despite my own religious beliefs, I felt ambiguous about the religious focus that emerged in these cases, as many assumptions about belief about God are left unaddressed. This was clearly a language and construct familiar to the chaplains who were comfortable using it, to the extent that they often took the lead in introducing it.

While Grossoehme captured the importance of how the child he worked with narrated her view of God in relation to her circumstances and setting, he was undoubtedly quite directive, introducing religious conundrums and supporting ritual; however, what was not explored was how this child's view correlated with the chaplain's own understanding of God. Hildebrand has a different perspective on how the parent presented her need through religious language. She stated, 'It is my goal to be aware of, and attentive to, feelings and needs that may be buried beneath a person's initial self-presentation as a person of faith.' While Grossoehme constructed a religious narrative within which to offer care, Hildebrand deconstructed religious views in order to address the parent's needs. With her own profiling, which included in the past being a Quaker, Hildebrand may have her own deconstructive agenda, implied when she uses the phrase, 'my goal was to get religion out of the way'. This could be a false dichotomy that prejudices her care of others.

Piderman demonstrates a similar model but seems to have an integrated approach that allows her to state:

I remember reaching deep inside to center myself in my belief that God is with us always, and perhaps especially in our deepest darkness. I wanted to be present with Angela and faithful to her in her darkness, but also to help her find what centered her.

With respect to the other chaplains, I found that Piderman captured a helpful blend of what may have been intended in the other cases, when she stated, 'My goals were to respect her, be attentive to her and offer compassion, but also to challenge her in a way that might open new doors to God's grace. I decided to offer her my perspective.' Piderman provided a platform for mutual respect so that both she and the patient could explore together their views and thoughts as a basis for discussion, rather than on the premise for the need to agree.

The chaplains have each demonstrated how their religious conceptual thinking, their grasp of biblical narrative and their ability to create a liturgical space can be key elements when an encounter has a religious dimension; however, these key elements need to be handled appropriately so that they contribute to the care of the parent or patient on their own terms.

A final observation and comment

An obvious, but nonetheless important, observation is that the parameters of pediatrics vary: from a United Kingdom perspective, Grossoehme and Piderman could be considered to lie outside the pediatric setting, simply because of the age range set for clinical practice. More striking is the overtly religious content of these cases. The selection of these religious encounters by the chaplains introduces another factor into each case study. Whether these are unusual or typical of the US spiritual and religious profile, what matters is how the chaplain responds. The level of repeat visits is more than in my own practice; not that I did not experience repeat visits, but rather my focus was more on responding to crisis. In Grossoehme's case, the level of care offered in the hope that further care could be provided in the future when the child's condition becomes critical could, in a different pediatric healthcare setting, be viewed as an indulgent use of time. This is not a criticism but an acknowledgement that fuller resources offer greater opportunity for long-term care.

I am acutely aware that I have made comments on colleagues who have each faced challenging circumstances and have been prepared to put themselves in an exposed place so that others can learn. I have the deepest respect and admiration for Grossoehme, Hildebrand and Piderman, and I thank them for the deep privilege of learning from them.

References

Bull, A. (2012) 'The insights gained from a portfolio of spiritual assessment tools used with hospitalised school-aged children to facilitate the delivery of spiritual care offered by the healthcare chaplain.' Unpublished dissertation. Glasgow: University of Glasgow Library.

Foucault, M. (1982) 'Afterword: The subject and power.' In H.L. Dreyfus and P. Rabinow (eds) *Michel Foucault: Beyond Structuralism and Hermeneutics.* Hemel Hempstead: The Harvester Press, 208–226.

O'Connor, T.S., O'Neill, K., Van Staalduinen, G., Meakes, E., Penner, C. and Davis, K. (2005) 'Not well known, used little and needed: Canadian chaplains' experiences of published spiritual assessment tools.' *Journal of Pastoral Care and Counsel 59,* 1–2, 97–107.

Chapter 5

Critical Response to Pediatric Case Studies

A Psychologist's Perspective

Sian Cotton

My responses to these case studies come from my vantage point as a clinical health psychologist. I spend most of my work time conducting pediatric health outcomes research and directing a complementary and integrative medicine program at a large academic health center. Much of my previous research has been in the area of spiritual coping of people with chronic conditions, particularly children/adolescents. As such, I have spent considerable time interviewing and surveying children/adolescents and their parents about the role that God and their faith plays in their illness, how they utilize religious or spiritual coping, and assessing spiritual struggles in relation to an illness. I have also worked closely on research with chaplain and medicine colleagues, and continue to learn the value of differing interdisciplinary perspectives and how we enrich each others' work by sharing our own perspectives. My reflections focus primarily on: (1) What chaplains do; (2) How chaplains think about what they do; and (3) Some thoughts on the role of case studies in informing research and the practice of chaplaincy in healthcare.

Case 1

Presented by Chaplain Grossoehme, the first case study is of a 12-year-old Euro-American girl, who has been living with cystic fibrosis (CF) since age 1 year and also with CF-related diabetes since age 4–5 years. With frequent inpatient hospitalizations and outpatient visits, including much missed school, Chaplain Grossoehme describes an ongoing relationship with LeeAnn (he has known her for 5 years), with the focus of his care being to 'build and maintain a pastoral relationship with LeeAnn…so that she would feel free to ask religious/existential questions as she grew older and/or her disease progressed'. He describes doing the following within the context of her care: (a) developing and maintaining the relationship; (b) utilizing secular interests to engage her in spiritual exploration (e.g. including play and drawing); (c) praying – though he is clear that he does not always pray just to 'distinguish' himself from other providers; (d) exploring her image of, and connection to, God; (e) discussing her use of spiritual coping resources; and (f) listening to her tell her story.

When considering how Chaplain Grossoehme's pastoral care contributed to LeeAnn's (and her family's) well-being and/or peace, it strikes me most that the visits from him provided LeeAnn with comfort and connection, as evidenced by her ongoing and open engagement with him and the reported positive affect during his visits. For a child with a chronic illness, indeed for any child, steady, consistent, positive relationships with trusted adults are critical for healthy development and attachment. Chaplain Grossoehme's regular presence was likely a source of positive strength for her, communicating active care and concern for her well-being. While we do not hear much about how the parents or other family members felt about the chaplain's presence, we might presume that they are comforted that LeeAnn has this professional contact to assist her with her isolation and coping during her hospitalizations. It was noticeable that Chaplain Grossoehme did not report routinely asking about LeeAnn's emotional functioning at each visit (though maybe he asked and just did not report on it).

Presumably, her emotional functioning and ability to cope with her stressors and situation are a key piece of information any chaplain would need to know.

In Chaplain Grossoehme's description of his work, he often states that relationship building is an outcome unto itself. This is an interesting question to ponder: Is the relationship *itself* the outcome or does the relationship help us to achieve our clinical, professional and spiritual 'outcomes' with a patient or family member? Clearly there is no correct answer. Chaplain Grossoehme described two primary chaplaincy issues: (a) isolation; and (b) relationship building and maintenance. While the establishment of this long-term trusting professional relationship is an important goal, particularly for a child with a life-shortening condition who has a great deal of burden and uncertainty in her life, I wonder what other issues could be explored now. For example, I was struck regarding the repeated theme of her isolation, that the isolation itself was not described as either a focus of treatment or a theme that was woven throughout. Rather, the focus was very forward projected, preparing her for when a crisis might come. I would suggest that a state of isolation, particularly from school and peers for a 12-year-old girl, is a developmental crisis unto itself and worthy of attention (whether this was in spiritual care or mental healthcare visits would depend in part on the team and her relationship to it). So, for example, inquiries such as the following could be appropriate: 'What is it like for you to be in hospital on your own so much? Do you feel disconnected from your family and friends? If so, how might God or prayer support you?' I was also curious that the topic of 'endings' specifically was not raised more with LeeAnn. For a child with over 100 surgeries and a life-shortening condition, exploring even a discharge from the hospital as an example of an ending would seem a ripe opportunity for discussing existential issues including transitions, endings and eventually death.

I admire Chaplain Grossoehme for raising the issue of a theoretically driven practice of chaplaincy. This is a critical point, and I believe that it is a very worthwhile conversation for the future of the field of healthcare chaplaincy. However, I do believe that drawing from theories from related disciplines (e.g. social work, nursing, psychology) in the absence of good theoretical chaplain models is a step in the right direction for the future of the discipline. For example, in the training of psychologists, we often have students describe a 'case/patient' from multiple theoretical perspectives and present related goals and treatment plans. So, for example, we could conceptualize LeeAnn from a family-systems or developmental perspective, with a focus on reducing her isolation and increasing her sense of connectedness; or from a cognitive-behavioral perspective, where we might identify negative cognitions as they impact her functioning and mood, and help adjust those cognitions; or a narrative-therapy perspective in which she would work on 'rewriting' her story in ways that would facilitate healthy adaptation to current struggles. In considering 'developing a theory of chaplaincy', as Chaplain Grossoehme suggests, I would strongly recommend borrowing from decades of theories from related disciplines while continuing to foster a core tenant arising from chaplaincy itself.

Case 2

Discussed by Chaplain Hildebrand, the second case study is of a pastoral relationship for a year and a half with Erica, the mother of a 2-year-old, Macy, who was an inpatient and undergoing intensive treatment for cancer. In her description, Chaplain Hildebrand describes 'witnessing', being a mindful listening presence and 'holding' Erica during their regular sessions. She also describes facilitating emotional expression (anger, sadness) and praying as part of her role. The case is very thoughtfully presented and conceptualized in a way that indicates great care in the chaplain's thoughtfulness regarding her work. Chaplain Hildebrand's descriptions, both of her work with Erica and how she interpreted her actions, are, from a psychology-theory perspective, psychodynamic, and they even draw from the theory of object relations. At one point the chaplain said she was trying to 'reach into Erica's life experience', expressing a depth of wanting to connect closely with Erica in order to understand her better and presumably assist her along a spiritual path.

It appears that the relationship that was established with Chaplain Hildebrand allowed Erica to go deeper and open up in significant ways for her healing. It is interesting to consider whether, in a shorter time frame with fewer visits, this relationship could have been established. She describes Erica's 'unmet spiritual needs' as being underneath the familiar religious-speak, and that she helped her articulate those needs at her own pace: 'It is my goal to be aware of, and attentive to, feelings and needs that may be buried beneath a person's initial self-presentation as a person of faith.' Chaplain Hildebrand wanted to convey that she was available to go beyond religious conversation to a deeper level. So a question for the reader: How much time does it take to develop deeper relationships for effective pastoral care? Can they be developed in a shorter-term, crisis-oriented model of care? This does raise the more general question about healthcare chaplaincy and different models of care, for example, a model that is more crisis oriented compared with a model based more in prevention and routine care inherent in the hospital stay.

Of note, Chaplain Hildebrand describes a sense of relief or clinical freedom knowing that social work was taking care of Erica's psychosocial goals, giving her the ability to let Erica lead where she wanted to go in the conversations. This raises another interesting clinical question about whether additional mental health or related disciplines are involved in the care of a particular patient, and if so, whether this changes the focus and the goals of the pastoral care.

The chaplain did spend appropriate energy on deeper issues such as loss, family, her past, coping and relationships, all having been opened up after the initial 'let's talk about God' theme that Erica was following. Interestingly, in the summary, Chaplain Hildebrand interprets Erica not initially talking to her about family and stressors as related to possible shame. An alternate explanation is that many people may not have a good model in their head about what they are 'supposed' to talk to a chaplain about, so they talk about God because that is what they think they are supposed to talk about. In much the same way, Erica maybe did not talk to the social workers about God because she didn't think she was 'supposed' to. This highlights a more general clinical point about informing patients up front about what the expectations of the chaplain's visit are, and what the space can hold.

The most fascinating quote to me was Chaplain Hildebrand saying that 'my goal was to get religion out of the way so that spiritual care could begin'. The researcher in me wants to know what her definition of 'spiritual care' is. (I presume we all may have very different definitions.) An area for inquiry might be: How do you define 'spiritual care'? What do you define as 'good spiritual care'? It seems that when Erica was done praying and talking about God, and started sharing about her family, Macy's illness and her substance use, the chaplain felt pleased that the work had finally begun.

The chaplain's clinical style of listening, rather than leading and not analyzing, is a Rogerian empathic listening approach that I believe underlies much of pastoral care and training. It is similar to the non-directive listening of many psychodynamic therapy approaches, and quite different than cognitive-behavioral or solution-focused therapies which are more goal oriented and involve giving concrete suggestions around behaviors and emotions. There is no right or wrong, just an interesting note for the field of chaplaincy to ponder the pros and cons of remaining primarily non-directive and focused on listening and/or witnessing rather than being more directly goal oriented.

Case 3

The case presented by Chaplain Piderman is of Angela, a 17-year-old girl, who was in a car accident in which she was left paralyzed. With little family or social support and limited coping resources, Angela was in a rehabilitation unit when the chaplain met her and began working with her to build rapport and understand her spiritual and religious landscape. As her goals, the chaplain states that she wants to 'be a sign of God's incarnational love' and to help Angela establish a relationship with God that would 'center and sustain her' when she was no longer in the hospital. She also describes that her role on the team is to 'conduct spiritual assessments and facilitate and/or provide spiritual care'.

Notably, and different from the other two pediatric cases, Chaplain Piderman describes using two spiritual assessment tools up front to help understand Angela's spiritual needs and resources. Though not stated, I would hope that these assessments were documented in the chart for the rest of the team to see. If they were, it suggests an interesting practice-based research opportunity, namely, gathering systematic data over time from these tools, that may be in electronic health records at various sites across the country, and utilizing these data to conduct outcomes research (e.g. one could examine level of spiritual resources as related to use of mental health services) or quality improvement initiatives.

Chaplain Piderman describes the many active and passive strategies she employed during her care of Angela: listening; sitting quietly while Angela processed emotions or cried; witnessing; helping guide Angela through difficult emotions; giving voice to Angela's negative emotions (i.e. the suffering); using Scripture as interpretation; assisting Angela in exploring her relationship with God and to the accident; discussing how she is coping; exploring spiritual struggles; praying with her; and working hand-in-hand with the interdisciplinary team both in treatment goal-setting and in discharge planning. Her interventions and clinical choices with Angela seem to be spot on, and seemingly allowed Angela to raise some very difficult questions. While not all questions were answered during the course of care, it does seem that critical existential issues and the use of spiritual coping strategies were raised and 'held' during the spiritual care provided. One area that might have been explored more, if given time and opportunity, are the issues around loss and abandonment by Angela's mother (and father) and how this might relate to her own losses via her accident, including her expressed feelings of abandonment by God. It strikes me that we did not hear much about her anger at her mother, particularly given the mother's decision to not care for Angela upon her release from the rehabilitation unit.

This was one of the most emotionally and spiritually powerful stories that I have ever read. Chaplain Piderman was viscerally able to communicate Angela's pain, her plight and journey, how this was witnessed, how the spiritual care transformed and assisted Angela, and even how she herself as a chaplain was moved by this relationship. I believe the powerful nature of storytelling via case presentations such as this gives voice to the stories that are being 'held' within the discipline of chaplaincy that may need to be shared, if not only to better understand the discipline and direction of chaplaincy both in past and present forms, but also to give voice to the needs and desires of the discipline growing into the future.

The important role of chaplains working within interdisciplinary teams is raised in this case. In particular, it is noted that on teams such as these, sometimes one provider can make progress with challenging issues when another provider cannot. We see a rich example of this when the psychologist and team are struggling with adherence issues and self-care with Angela, whereas the chaplain is able to work with her successfully to move her through these issues. It also raises the complex issue of the intertwining relationships between chaplaincy and various mental health disciplines (e.g. social work, psychology) and how these various clinical relationships relate (and sometimes overlap) with each other to achieve optimal outcomes and support for patients and families.

Chaplain Piderman provides a very nice case example of using other theoretical and developmental work for her case conceptualization, and to assist with guiding treatment. She also utilizes recent research on quality of life and adjustment of patients with spinal cord injuries to inform her thinking about Angela and her long-term adjustment. The chaplain's ability to reflect on her own feelings and her own spiritual beliefs lead to a deep, thoughtful understanding that I believe ultimately benefited Angela in her care.

Conclusion

In conclusion, these three pediatric chaplain case studies raise many complex and thought-provoking issues for the field: developing a theory of chaplaincy and/or utilizing existing theories; interprofessional teams and relationships with other mental health and social service providers; the use of research to inform practice; incorporating spiritual assessment screening tools; different models of chaplaincy care; directive versus non-directive chaplaincy care; and many others. The capacity of case studies as a means to generate ideas for research and quality improvement initiatives in chaplaincy is not to be underestimated. As additional chaplain case studies are reported, it is akin to 'theme generation' in qualitative research, where consistent and divergent themes are identified and then followed by rigorous and informed studies that are designed to flush out critical ideas or questions for the discipline. The ultimate goal, of course, is to improve the quality of chaplaincy care being provided in order to better the health and well-being of the people and communities we serve.

Part 2
Psychiatric Case Studies

Steve Nolan

The idea that spiritual care can be delivered regardless of training is common within healthcare (Ronaldson 1997; McSherry 2001, 2006; Wright and Neuberger 2012). Without question, nurses 'hold a unique position in the delivery of patient care' (McSherry 2001, p.109); equally, many nurses 'recognise that attending to the spiritual needs of patients enhances the overall quality of nursing care' (McSherry and Jamieson 2011, p.1765). However, 'the majority of [UK] nurses' report they feel ill-equipped 'to support and effectively meet their patients' spiritual needs' (McSherry and Jamieson 2011, p.1763). The fact is that delivering spiritual care demands not only a particular mix of knowledge and skills, but a high degree of subtlety in applying that mix.

The case presented by Chaplain Ratcliffe is a particularly good example of the way an experienced chaplain is able, subtlety, to use her knowledge and skills to therapeutic effect. Chaplain Ratcliffe admits to knowing very little about Nigerian beliefs about witches, so she felt ill-prepared when called to help Yesuto, a Nigerian man in his early thirties troubled by his belief in witchcraft. Yesuto had a history of depression with episodes of psychosis and, while he described himself as a Christian, he took little strength from his faith, describing himself as a *bad* Christian. When he met Chaplain Ratcliffe, Yesuto catalogued the many ways in which he thought he had fallen short in his religious practice, and he told her that his illness was due to the fact that he had been 'bewitched' by an evil witch from his home in Nigeria.

Handicapped by her lack of specific knowledge, Chaplain Ratcliffe's work with Yesuto illustrates the way her training as a mental health chaplain equipped her to improvise, combining a person-centred approach that places a high value on the individual's experience and subjective reality, with a willingness to explore his belief system in a way that encourages him to question his beliefs in a safe and supported way. In this work, Chaplain Ratcliffe draws on her personal experience of cultural vulnerability and awareness of the pitfalls of cultural misunderstanding, and makes a strong case for the importance of cultural competence in healthcare settings.

Like Chaplain Grossoehme in his case study, Chaplain Ratcliffe emphasizes skilful listening as a central part of what a chaplain does. She makes clear that she is not a trained counsellor/therapist; nonetheless, she demonstrates how a chaplain's spiritual care can be informed by the person-centred approach of Carl Rogers and the skills of Socratic questioning, as developed within cognitive behavioural therapy. In her work with Yesuto, Chaplain Ratcliffe both listens actively, with empathy and without judgement, and uses skilful questioning to enable him constructively to address his own beliefs. What becomes apparent, through the process of listening and questioning, is that a significant proportion of what troubled Yesuto was sociocultural and religious rather than simply psychiatric, and that his psychiatric needs were being compounded by cultural misunderstanding on the part of his healthcarers. In this case, what makes the difference is not the good intentions of a well-meaning healthcarer, but the knowledge, skills and experience of a trained chaplain who understands the nature of belief and how it operates to construct an individual's sociocultural frame of reference or world view.

The distinctive qualities chaplains bring to their work is highlighted in the case presented by Chaplain Swift, who draws attention to a unique risk healthcare chaplains face. This risk arises from the fact that chaplains are normally religious figures, and as such they carry a set of associations and connotations, both negative and positive. Specifically, the patient in this case assumed that anything she shared with a priest would be treated as sacrosanct. On that basis, June assumed that she could both speak openly about her life and honestly about her ongoing wish to commit suicide, and that these things would not be shared with other hospital staff, even though she might deceive her care team about her plans. Such an assumption would not have been made in relation to any other healthcare professional, and clearly it posed considerable ethical and professional questions, not the least being a perennial question faced by chaplains about whether or not their trust is being manipulated by those for whom they are caring. Agreeing to accompany June to her meeting with psychiatrists and be her support placed Chaplain Swift in the familiar, but uncomfortable, professional space that healthcare chaplains frequently occupy: employed to be part of a multidisciplinary care team, yet standing apart from it and alongside a patient whose true motivations cannot be known for certain. In this case, which occurred when he was a relatively inexperienced chaplain, Chaplain Swift reflects frankly on how he dealt with the situation. In the process, he demonstrates how even historical cases can yield important learning in reflective practice, and he highlights how this case underlines the need for thorough professional training for all chaplains, whether full- or part-time, and one might add, voluntary.

The centrality of the chaplain's unique identity is an important theme running through this case. In this case, June was apprehensive that she might be judged (and punished) for her attempted suicide and condemned for her homosexuality. In her younger days, June had had mixed experiences of chaplains, but once she had clarified with Chaplain Swift what sort of chaplain he would be for her, she felt able to express her theological question, which concerned whether God would punish her for who she was and what she had done. Perhaps what gave June the freedom to put her questions to him was her understanding that chaplains occupy a place apart, and given her previous experience that some chaplains were *genuinely* interested in helping people, she felt enabled to confide in someone she perceived to be of the religious institution (and could bring sacraments) and yet, simultaneously, apart from it (i.e. would not judge her in a way she might have expected).

Like Chaplain Swift, Chaplain Zollfrank places a high value on autonomy. At the heart of her case is an ethical dilemma that is concerned with supporting a young man from the Dominican Republic to make autonomous, adult choices about his sexual identity. Nate's struggle had threatened his life, since he had made several failed attempts at suicide. His struggle was compounded by his cultural background and his religious beliefs. The ethical dilemma his case poses is whether a chaplain should seek, through supportive education, to empower a person to make autonomous choices when those choices risk deepening the sense of isolation that led him to attempt suicide but, equally, could lead to a sense of personal authenticity that may enable him to overcome his isolation.

As in the case presented by Chaplain Ratcliffe, culture plays a significant part in the chaplaincy encounter with Nate. Both Nate and Chaplain Zollfrank are immigrants to the US; both share certain experiences in common, in particular, the renegotiating of identity in a context different from their culture and families of origin. However, there are significant points of difference: age, gender, sexual orientation and denominational differences being perhaps the most pertinent. These differences pose a challenge to the chaplaincy encounter, particularly when that encounter is motivated by beneficence, which can sometimes be difficult to distinguish from paternalism.

Chaplain Zollfrank works closely with the interdisciplinary team of her institution. In this, she adopts a supportive role that frequently manifests in terms of education: normalizing certain of Nate's experiences, for example, his struggle with the difference between his values and those of his parents, or explaining that he was not alone in finding certain religious/spiritual attitudes helpful or unhelpful; and offering alternative ways of understanding human sexuality and sexual development, again explaining differences between the teachings of religious denominations. As such, her approach presents a contrasting style of chaplaincy to others in this book, one that is more directive than most. Readers will be interested in Chaplain Zollfrank's comments about the possibility of Nate's compliance with her and her views about the benefits of involving a Roman Catholic priest in supporting Nate.

Several cases in this book illustrate how training in counselling/psychotherapy, even to a limited degree, may inform chaplains' work. Both respondents to the cases in this section have some degree of dual training. Graeme D. Gibbons, a chaplain who also practises as a psychoanalytical self-psychologist, highlights how the figure of the witch, in Chaplain Ratcliffe's case, could be read as a metaphor for those witch-like figures (archetypes?) that haunt the psyches of many Westerners. He uses Chaplain Swift's case to draw attention to the chaplain's role as a theologian, identifying and providing answers to genuine theological questions. And, following Brandchaft, he names as 'pathological accommodation' a process chaplains should watch for in their own practice: the subtle (or otherwise) pressure to conform to the expectations of the other (Brandchaft 2010).

Warren Kinghorn, a psychiatrist with theological training, begins his response with pertinent observations about what he describes as the 'complex interweaving of spiritual matters into the fabric of mental health problems' and the difficulties chaplains can face in negotiating their 'correlatively complex relationship with other members of the multidisciplinary care team'. He presents his response as commentary on how each case supports patients torn between their formative religious tradition, the normative expectations of the medical care team and their own evolving sense of personal identity. From his dual perspective, Kinghorn highlights potential hazards of dual qualification. For example, a chaplain may be sensitized, by religious training, to the way the medical model can pathologize a person's religious experience, yet they may miss the way they use their psychological training to pathologize the same person's religious belief. This is perhaps one of the risks of serving in the place of liminality.

References

Brandchaft, B., Doctors, S. and Sorter, D. (2010) *Toward an Emancipatory Psychoanalysis: Brandchaft's Intersubjective Vision.* New York, NY: Routledge.

McSherry, W. (2001) 'Spiritual crisis? Call a nurse.' In H. Orchard (ed) *Spirituality in Health Care Contexts.* London: Jessica Kingsley Publishers, 107–117.

McSherry, W. (2006) *Making Sense of Spirituality in Nursing and Health Care Practice: An Interactive Approach* (2nd edn). London: Jessica Kingsley Publishers.

McSherry, W. and Jamieson, S. (2011) 'An online survey of nurses' perceptions of spirituality and spiritual care.' *Journal of Clinical Nursing 20,* 11–12, 1757–1767.

Ronaldson, S. (ed) (1997) *Spirituality: The Heart of Nursing.* Melbourne: Ausmed Publications.

Wright, S. and Neuberger, J. (2012) 'Why spirituality is essential for nurses.' *Nursing Standard 26,* 40, 19–21.

Chapter 6

'I am frightened to close my eyes at night in case the witch comes to me in my sleep'

– Yesuto, a Nigerian man in his early thirties troubled by his belief in witchcraft

Rosie Ratcliffe

Introduction

I received a call from a ward asking me to visit with a male patient who was religious and having fearful thoughts. I was told that the client's name was Yesuto and that he had particular beliefs about witchcraft that were causing him great distress and interfering with his treatment. It was explained that these beliefs had been an ongoing problem since his admission a week earlier.

Yesuto was a Nigerian man in his early thirties. He was educated to secondary school level in a private boarding school in Nigeria and had been in the UK from the age of 18 years. The only detail I was given regarding his diagnosis was that he had a long history of depression with episodes of psychosis; however, although his diagnoses formed the context and backdrop of my meeting, it did not figure overtly in my discussion with the client. Yesuto had been in hospital for a week prior to his referral to the Spiritual and Pastoral Care Service. While it is not possible to reveal the exact ward to which he was admitted, I can reveal that he was on one of what, at the time, were termed the 'Specialist' units.

The case took place in 2004, when I was serving as an ordained Anglican Chaplain to the National and Specialist Wards at the Bethlem Hospital (these included eating disorders, mother and baby, self-harm, psychosis and affective disorders, among others). I had been ordained around three and a half years prior to taking up this post and had served a three-year stipendiary curacy. Prior to my ordination, I had also served as a mental health lay chaplain for three years at both Warlingham Park and Bethlem hospitals. It was here that I received my initial mental health training, which involved close clinical supervision and the development of self-reflective practice. I should add that I am not a trained counsellor or therapist.

Although I was raised in England from the age of 6 months, I was born in Baghdad and am of Assyrian origin. My upbringing was, therefore, steeped in Assyrian culture and I believe that my personal experience of the impact of culture upon beliefs and upbringing did have a bearing on this case.

Unfortunately, it was not possible to trace the person concerned to ask their permission to publish the details of the encounter; therefore, for matters of confidentiality, and in order to protect the anonymity of this person, I have withheld a number of details about the case and changed others. Since the client came from the continent of Africa and was also a devout Christian, I have given him the pseudonym Yesuto, which, I am informed, translates as 'belongs to Jesus'. While the case took place in 2004, I have referred to the notes that I kept at the time; also, I have used the case study for training purposes on a number of occasions, which has kept it fresh in my mind.

Case study
History of relationship

As I made my way to the ward, I recognized that I was quite nervous about this referral. 'What do I know about witches, and how on earth am I supposed to help?' I was completely uncertain as to the best way to approach this situation, and since this was a referral from the medical team, I felt that 'all eyes are on me', so to speak. I decided the best way forward was simply to meet the client 'where he was at'. This meant that my priority was to work with complete empathic understanding, that is, to try to understand what the client was going through, from his perspective (Rogers 1980, 1986). This approach meant placing a high value on the experience of the individual and on the importance of his subjective reality.

I was introduced to Yesuto as the chaplain by a member of staff, and we were given a private room for the consultation. Yesuto was initially withdrawn and reticent to speak, and since he was so disengaged, I needed to build a rapport with him in order to achieve some level of meaningful communication. I began by saying that I had been asked to visit him by the medical staff.

I recognize that such an approach may have been interpreted in a number of ways. It is possible Yesuto could have read the direct communication between me and the staff in a threatening, even judgemental, way; however, this was not a social setting, and it was not appropriate to begin with superficial niceties. It was also important to begin the encounter in an open, honest and authentic way, ensuring there was no dissonance between my words and intentions. Furthermore, years of experience as a chaplain have taught me to become very conscious of rapport building; it is not all about the words we use. Usually, we create and maintain rapport unconsciously and instinctively through matching non-verbal signals with the other person, including body positioning, body movements, eye contact, facial expressions and tone of voice; however, although rapport building happens unconsciously through non-verbal communication, it is possible to make conscious use of the technique

(Winbolt 2011). I was, therefore, very mindful of my body language and tone of voice, ensuring that I spoke softly in order to convey empathy, all the while maintaining eye contact in order to match myself with the client.

I then asked Yesuto whether he thought there was any way that I could help or support him. Yesuto began by speaking to me about his faith, and it was not long before he seemed quite at ease, speaking freely and openly. It became very clear during the course of our conversation that Yesuto had harsh religious beliefs that left him feeling inadequate and sinful. As I listened to him, I began to point out aspects of Jesus' teaching and sections of the Bible that speak of unconditional love, acceptance and forgiveness. He responded by saying that he had 'forgotten' about these teachings, and to each revelation and biblical example of love and acceptance that I gave he kept repeating 'that's true, that's true'. Below is a verbatim of the exchange:

> *Chaplain:* My name is Rosie and staff called me and asked me to visit you. (*Yesuto says nothing and simply nods. I pause for a little while and then say.*) You must be having a difficult time at the moment. (*Yesuto again says nothing and simply nods. I again pause for a while before saying.*) Do you think there is anything I can do to help you?
>
> *Yesuto:* (*hesitantly*) I am a Christian.
>
> *Chaplain:* You know it wouldn't matter to me even if you weren't a Christian. I am here to help anyone and everyone, regardless of whether or not they are a Christian.
>
> *Yesuto:* (*Nods and then says more confidently.*) I was brought up a Christian and always went to church every Sunday, but I am a very bad Christian now. I don't go to church; I haven't been to church for a long time. I don't pray enough or read the Bible enough. I am trying to read the Bible here in hospital, but I am finding it difficult. I am such a bad person and a bad Christian. I am [a] sinner…all of my suffering is deserved.

It is possible that, in assuring Yesuto that I was a priest, open to anyone and everyone, regardless of whether or not they had a faith, I may have helped him relax into the conversation. Yesuto was so full of self-condemnation and guilt due to his lapsed Christian practices that he may have thought I, too, would judge him harshly. Although I am well aware that there are numerous ways in which religion is advantageous for psychological and physical health – for example, in bolstering feelings of hope, optimism, self-esteem, belonging and meaning – I had worked in mental health for long enough to immediately recognize that here was a brand of religion and Christianity that was detrimental to mental well-being (see Kim-Goh 1993; Pfeifer 1994; Trenholm, Trent and Compton 1998; Nicholls 2002; Ukst-Margetic and Margetic 2005; Dein et al. 2010). When religious beliefs become dogmatic, inflexible and a burden to people, instead of reducing anxiety, they can be damaging. Here I felt on familiar ground and it was very clear that Yesuto's beliefs left him guilt-ridden and feeling inadequate and sinful. After Yesuto catalogued the areas where he felt he fell short in religious practice, I responded:

> Chaplain: What about those parts of the Bible where Jesus teaches about unconditional love and forgiveness? The Prodigal Son, for example, he more or less says to his father 'I want you dead' when he asks for his share of the inheritance. He squanders all the money and yet his father *runs* to greet him. There is no mention of his sin or what he did wrong. He is embraced without any question.

> Yesuto: (*nods*) That's true.

> Chaplain: There's also the Samaritan woman. She had a questionable past with five husbands, and Jesus doesn't condemn her.

> Yesuto: (*nods*) That's true…that's true. I had forgotten about these teachings. Thank you for reminding me.

Yesuto and I spoke a little more about religion and faith, and I pointed out that since he was unwell and in hospital he might try to be gentle with himself and to give himself permission *not* to read the Bible, or pray, unless it was helping him. I said to Yesuto that if he had broken every bone in his body, and was lying on a hospital bed in a general hospital, he might feel less inclined to judge himself for not reading the Bible or being in church.

I then reflected back on another point that Yesuto had initially made, that his 'suffering [was] deserved', and I asked him whether he would like to say a little bit more about that. Yesuto responded by telling me that he was unwell because he had been 'bewitched' by an evil witch in Nigeria. He was extremely tense and distressed as he talked to me, and in order to understand more about his situation I asked a question:

Chaplain: Yesuto, why has this witch chosen to 'target' you?

Yesuto: There are so many witches in Nigeria, and they are malicious, they have no compassion. They are evil, and they like to inflict suffering and death on people. It is what they do. That is their work. I am so frightened. I am frightened for my baby. I think that he is going to die when he is 8 years old. The doctors and staff keep telling me I am sick and that, if I take my medication, I will get better and I will no longer be scared of witches. I cannot sleep. I am frightened to close my eyes at night in case the witch comes to me in my sleep. I am so tired, so tired and scared. I don't know how much longer I can go on.

Yesuto's body language, his facial expression and, in particular, the way in which he was sitting, appeared strained and uneasy. He told me that he felt utterly powerless because he had no way of countering the effects of the magic spells that were cast over him. He kept repeating that he was afraid to close his eyes at night in case the witch visited him in his sleep.

That Yesuto felt physically and emotionally threatened, and that these feelings were very real, was highly evident. He was communicating intense feelings very openly, and I did not wish to minimize or rationalize these distressing feelings in any way. As a chaplain, I knew it was paramount that Yesuto had the space to express these feelings, and I simply listened, actively, with empathy, suspending all judgement, simply meeting Yesuto at his point of contact, and my opening question, 'Why has this witch chosen to target you?' reflected this. I did not contradict his current perceptions and experiences.

Yesuto went on to tell me that his parents were visiting from Nigeria, and that they too were convinced that his illness was the result of witchcraft. They were telling him not to take the medication prescribed by the doctors, as this would simply aggravate the situation and make him more ill. To make matters worse, Yesuto's wife had also recently given birth to their first child, and his parents were warning him not to love his son too much. Loving a child too much simply ensured that the child would die.

As I listened to Yesuto, he said that he was greatly relieved that I was taking his beliefs seriously. All the medical staff he had encountered so far had dismissed his fears and beliefs, telling him that he was simply ill. They kept reiterating that if he took his medication, his fear about witches would disappear. While I had not spoken with the psychiatrist responsible for Yesuto's care, the conversation that I had had with the nurses prior to meeting him confirmed that the staff considered his beliefs about witches to be a symptom of his illness. It was clear that by listening to Yesuto with empathic understanding and without judgement, he felt heard and understood.

When Yesuto finished speaking, I was most acutely aware of his fear and discomfort. I did not think consciously about what I was going to say to him, it was an intuitive response. Uppermost in my mind was the need to find some way of relieving his fear and terror of this witch.

> *Chaplain:* Yesuto, can you tell me whether you have felt any safer since you were admitted to hospital?
>
> *Yesuto: (faintly)* Yes, I feel a bit safer.
>
> *Chaplain: (I reflect this answer back to Yesuto.)* So since you have been admitted to hospital you feel safer; safer than you did at home?
>
> *Yesuto:* Yes, I feel a bit safer.
>
> *Chaplain:* And do you think you have felt a little bit better since you have been here?
>
> *Yesuto:* Yes, maybe, a little bit. I feel better here than I did at home. I was going out of my mind at home.
>
> *Chaplain:* So since you came to hospital a week ago you feel a bit safer and a little bit better.

Yesuto: Yes.

Chaplain: And I know that at times the staff have given you medication to help you sleep. Have the tablets worked and helped you at all?

Yesuto: Yes, a little.

Chaplain: OK, so since you have been in hospital, you have felt a little safer and a little bit better…at times.

Yesuto: (*nods*) Yes.

Chaplain: Well, I don't know very much about the witches in Nigeria. I only know what you have told me and you have been telling how very powerful they are, and that their power can reach you here in England; but, you know, if you feel even a tiny bit safer, and at times even a tiny bit better in hospital, then I, as an outsider, have to question the power of these witches back in Nigeria. How is it that their power can't penetrate the walls of this hospital making you feel even worse?

Yesuto was visibly startled by what I had said. His body language and demeanour changed from being hunched and cowering to sitting more upright with eyes wide. He was more animated and awake. After a moment of silence I spoke again:

Chaplain: Yesuto, have you ever wondered why it is that here in England we don't seem to have any problems with witches? Do you know any powerful, tormenting English witches?

Yesuto was quiet for a time and then he shook his head. 'No,' he said quietly. Yesuto and I talked more around this new perspective and he began to gradually make a connection between differing cultural beliefs and his fears. There was a more or less immediate, positive result from this approach.

Since the idea that his child would die at the age of 8 years was also creating high levels of anxiety, I then moved on to address this issue. I began by asking Yesuto to tell me more about his fears surrounding his newborn child and why he thought his parents were warning him not to love his child too much. Yesuto told me that his parents and grandparents had always taught him that loving a child too much would increase the likelihood of the child suffering harm in some way. I asked Yesuto whether he thought such beliefs were a result of parents trying to protect themselves from the emotional trauma of losing a child in countries where child mortality rates were high. This was something that Yesuto was again willing to consider, and it helped him to re-examine his parents' viewpoint, which he was struggling with, especially since he was overwhelmed with love for his newborn child. When we ended this particular discussion, I asked Yesuto about his own childhood. I wondered if anything significant had happened to him when he was 8 years old:

> *Chaplain:* Yesuto, what was it like for you growing up in Nigeria? Do you have happy memories of your childhood?
>
> *Yesuto:* Yes, I had a wonderful life at home in my village and with my family.

Yesuto told me about some of his childhood memories.

> *Chaplain: (After some minutes I asked him.)* What happened to you when you were 8 years old?
>
> *Yesuto:* My parents sent me away to boarding school.
>
> *Chaplain:* And what was that like for you?
>
> *Yesuto:* It was terrible. I was so unhappy. The teachers were so strict and they would punish us. I remember crying myself to sleep. I used to beg my parents to take me home, but they said it was important that I stay at the school. I had no friends and felt very lonely.

Yesuto spoke to me in more detail about his unhappy experiences at the school and of the trauma of returning to the school after each vacation. I paused for a while:

> *Chaplain:* Yesuto, did you notice how we started off by speaking about your fears for your child and your thoughts around him dying when he is 8 years old?
>
> *Yesuto: (nods)* Yes.

Chaplain: Well, look where we have ended up. We have just been talking about your very unhappy experiences when you were 8 years old. You experienced a terrible trauma when you were eight and it has stayed with you. Do you think there could be a connection between your past experiences and your fear for your child's future?

Yesuto: Maybe…maybe…I just never thought about it like that before.

Yesuto was relatively 'Westernized', but his cultural beliefs were constantly being reinforced by his parents who were visiting him from Nigeria. We discussed this together, and he told me that their visits always left him feeling more distressed and anxious. We therefore talked about various strategies and boundaries that he could put in place until they returned home.

Before I left, I prayed a prayer of protection for him, his child and his family, and since I worked part-time and would not be at work for a few days, I assured him that I would come back and see him. Although I did meet with Yesuto a further three or four times, the most important aspect of my work was carried out in that first visit. Yesuto was soon engaging more fully with the medical team as his fears dissipated more and more and, within a matter of weeks, he was discharged.

Discussion

Assessment

A number of problems were presenting with this client. First, the 'fear' that Yesuto was experiencing. He believed he had no way of protecting himself from someone whose power was unlimited and far reaching. Secondly, Yesuto's feelings of religious inadequacy were also causing him a great amount of distress. His very fixed and negative interpretation of Christianity, with its focus on sin and personal shortcomings, was causing him to be guilt ridden. Rather than his faith being a source of comfort and support, it merely compounded his suffering. In addition, Yesuto had concerns for his newborn child, who did not seem to be in immediate danger, but who, nevertheless, appeared to be destined to die at the age of 8 years. Finally, Yesuto's parents were exacerbating his problems by reinforcing his beliefs that his illness was a result of a witch in Nigeria and also by encouraging him not to love his child 'too much'.

Obviously, working in a mental health setting, I had met clients who were delusional, and in this particular case, too, I was open to the possibility that the client I was about to meet may have been suffering from delusions. However, my initial assessment of Yesuto, once I was introduced to him, was that, although he was shy and withdrawn, he was quite rational and capable of engaging intelligently in conversation. It soon became very apparent to me that an aspect of the problem that was presenting here was not a psychiatric one, but rather a sociocultural and religious one.

As an Assyrian growing up in England, I have personal experience of the important role that culture plays in a person's life. I also have an appreciation of the fact that people from different cultures are vulnerable to misunderstanding. Discrimination comes in many different forms, and sometimes even treating everyone the same, as unintentional as it might be, can be discriminatory. Glossing over differences, and thinking we are all the same, can create difficulties and misunderstandings. An understanding of cultural awareness is crucial in a healthcare setting where the aim is not just to accept or understand people, but to help and support them.

Of course, delivering mental health services to diverse populations is complex and multifaceted, and it is, therefore, vital that staff have an understanding of the roles culture and spirituality play with respect to illness and behaviour. As Cox argues:

> If mental health services in a multicultural society are to become more responsive to 'user' needs then eliciting this 'religious history' with any linked spiritual meanings should be a routine component

of a psychiatric assessment, and of preparing a more culturally sensitive 'care plan'. (Cox 1996, p.158; see also Dein 2004)

Awolalu (1975) underscores how religion is a fundamental – perhaps the most important – influence in the life of most Africans; yet its essential principles are too often unknown to non-Africans who, therefore, make themselves constantly liable to misunderstand the African world view and beliefs. Religion enters into every aspect of the life of Africans, and one of the most potent African superstitions is the belief in witchcraft. Most Africans believe witches are real, active beings that act to influence, intervene and alter the course of human life for good or ill. In this respect, witchcraft is accepted as a mode of explanation, perception and interpretation of life, events, nature and reality (Bannerman-Richter 1982; Palmer 2010). African scholar Aylward Shorter writes that belief in witchcraft is so pervasive that 'at the popular level the African believer is often more engrossed in the identification of human sources of evil, and in counteracting them, than in the acknowledgement and worship of superior forces of good' (cited in Agang 2009). This fear of sorcery within African Christianity is an old problem with a growing resurgence in modern Africa, a resurgence that has found its way into African communities in the West. In the UK, the recent killings of children Kristy Bamu, Victoria Klimbie and 'Adam' (the name given to the beheaded torso of a child found in the Thames in 2001) witness to this resurgence (Agang 2009; La Fontaine 2012). This demonstrates that Africans today continue to hold beliefs derived from the traditional cosmologies, and can apply these to everyday life, even when they live in cities. In this respect religious world views do not necessarily diminish with formal education (Ellis and ter Haar 2004). An important and crucial concept of cultural competence thus involves the incorporation of cultural ideologies and ethnocultural factors on the assessment and treatment of clients.

Although, when I met Yesuto, I was not aware of the sociocultural belief in witches among Africans, or of its prevalence, through popular culture I had heard of the extraordinary power that witch doctors in

Africa were believed to carry, and in my mind I equated the two. Since, due to my own upbringing, I was acutely aware of the impact of culture upon beliefs and behaviour, I was able to interact with Yesuto in a culturally sensitive way.

Interventions and outcomes

In meeting Yesuto, my primary approach was simply to listen and to support him through this difficult period. I had no prior in-depth knowledge or direct experience of Nigerian culture. Neither had I ever had an encounter with a client (or anyone else) that had a belief in witches.

Yesuto told me that his initial aloofness and disinterest in speaking to me was caused by a sense of discouragement. He had tried to engage with the medical staff regarding his beliefs, and these had been dismissed as symptoms of his illness. Giving Yesuto the opportunity to express his faith and religious beliefs, important aspects of his inner life, helped to build rapport and open up channels of communication, understanding and trust. Most importantly, when Yesuto moved on to speak to me about his belief in witches I did not, initially, attempt to counter or challenge his world view; I simply listened with empathy.

Empathy is one of the central dimensions of the therapeutic relationship. It is neither a response, nor a series of responses, but rather a continuing 'process' of 'being with' the client (Mearns and Thorne 1996, pp.39–40). Mearns and Thorne state that empathy should not be confused with sympathy. Whereas sympathy comes from feeling compassionately moved by the experience of another, and maybe even sharing in it, empathy requires the much more complex and delicate process of stepping into another person's shoes and seeing the world though the other person's eyes without, however, losing touch with one's own reality (Mearns and Thorne 1996, pp.26–27). Listening, too, is a very powerful tool and an important communication skill, and it is harder, and rarer, than a lot of people think: giving people time to talk, making appropriate eye contact, being physically still and relaxed, and not interrupting honours the client's emotional experience. It reflects an empathy that allows them space to express and release feelings that may be preventing them from moving forward (see, for example, Wagner 2006; Hick and Bien 2008).

After listening to Yesuto, and having assessed for myself that he appeared quite rational, since I knew little about African beliefs about witches, I was interested to learn from him. I therefore spent some time talking to him about this aspect of his life and experience. In this respect, the dialogue between us was one of fact finding. If I was going to help him, then I needed to understand more about the problem.

Talking to Yesuto about his beliefs, and his view of the world from his cultural perspective, gave him the opportunity and space to inform and teach me about his culture. This approach allowed for the development of trust within the encounter, and meant that he was not defensive but open to listening to what I had to say. Trust is one of the most important constructs within psychology for explaining interpersonal functioning and the outcomes of interactions (Marshall and Serran 2004), and other than their personality, knowledge and experience, therapists have very few tools at their disposal, unlike medical doctors. A therapist/chaplain, therefore, needs to use their personality in a way that fosters warmth and open communication in an endeavour to build trust. Indeed, Yesuto's initial aloofness may well have been a defensive mechanism and a form of self-protection from the persistent comments of staff that his fears were imaginary and merely a symptom of his illness.

Such an open and honest dialogue about his culture was enabled, both through the rapport that I had built up with Yesuto and also through my opening question, 'Why has this witch chosen to target you?' With this question I made no attempt to rationalize his beliefs, and because, at this point, I had put aside my own way of experiencing and perceiving reality, the process of empathic understanding with him was strengthened (Mearns and Thorne 1996, pp.39–40). This was a very different approach to that of the staff, who repeatedly told Yesuto that his beliefs were simply a symptom of his illness.

Since Yesuto felt unsafe and powerless, he was getting no rest or respite, either physical or mental. It was, therefore, important that this issue be addressed first and foremost. Therefore, as is the case with cognitive behavioural therapy, I focused on the 'here and now' and concentrated on trying to help him change his fearful thoughts by introducing a different perspective. The impact was an almost immediate improvement in his state of mind. With a change in his thoughts, there was a change in his feelings.

Our discussions over the subsequent visits, during a period of 3 weeks until he was finally discharged, centred mainly on the Christian teaching. Here again, I kept reinforcing the importance of focusing on love and acceptance, and trying to maintain a healthy balance in his thinking rather than distorting the Christian message with an overemphasis on sin and personal shortcomings. My aim was to help Yesuto to become much more conscious of his unhelpful thinking patterns and the negative things that he said to himself.

Further perspectives

This case study is a good example of how sociocultural beliefs impact upon a person's well-being. The sociocultural belief in witches holds a prominent place in the spirituality and religiosity of some cultures, and Yesuto's psychiatric condition was complicated by his religious and spiritual beliefs. He was obviously depressed and needed medical help; unfortunately, his belief in witches created a barrier between him and the medical team who were trying to help him. As far as the medical team were concerned, if he took his medication, then his fear about witches would go away. All he needed to do was to keep taking the medication, and eventually he would see sense. Unfortunately, that approach created relationship and communication problems between the staff and the client, compounding the client's suffering and sense of isolation. There are examples from the USA which demonstrate that gross errors in diagnosing, and grossly inappropriate services and interventions, have resulted from such cultural misunderstandings (Cuéllar and Paniagua 2000, p.xxvi). It is important that we avoid pathologizing, dismissing or ignoring the religious or spiritual experiences of clients.

Dein (2004) underscores the problems of countertransference, where mental health professionals become angered by patients with religious convictions, arguing that they hold 'primitive' and repressive beliefs that may be detrimental to mental health. He notes that such professionals may ask themselves how religious patients adhere to their belief systems in the absence of 'empirical' evidence. Greenberg and Witztum (1991) suggest that therapists may react to such emotions in a number of ways; in particular, they may ignore cultural influences or tensions and simply treat the patient as though they belong to their own cultural group. The psychiatrist who referred Yesuto to the chaplain felt that his fears and beliefs were 'irrational' and quite obviously a symptom of his illness. He was, therefore, referred to the chaplain, as the member of the multidisciplinary team (MDT) who is perhaps better equipped to deal with the ineffable and thus, perhaps, the irrational.

I, however, did not approach the problem in a way which suggested that his beliefs were wrong or misguided. The question I posed, 'Do you know of any English witches?' may seem intended to show him the error of his ways. It was *not*, in fact, motivated by a desire to change his beliefs, but actually to work with his belief system; it encouraged him to question his beliefs in a safe and supported way. His heightened emotional state and sense of fear had, up to this point, meant that his focus of attention was much narrowed and he was unable to consider alternative realities (LeDoux 1998). The question prompted the client to investigate his beliefs and to consider alternatives (Beck *et al.* 1979) and, by looking for evidence of his beliefs in countries other than his own, he was able to develop a more flexible and helpful way of thinking about the world, and thus work towards more helpful thought processes (Meyer 2011, p.47). I may have asked the question, but the actual exploration of the problem and the thought process was the work of the client himself (Beck *et al.* 1979). He challenged and altered his own thoughts; I was simply the catalyst. Yesuto was very quickly able to work out for himself that different cultures hold different beliefs and the way those beliefs are acted out and experienced in society differ accordingly. The question allowed him to put the problem in some kind of perspective, and it also helped him to understand that there were different dimensions to the problem. It ultimately gave him the ability to reframe or reinterpret a situation that had previously seemed uncontrollable.

Psychosis and depression are symptoms of a deep need, and in this particular case the client's fear of witches was seen as a manifestation of those symptoms. However, because a trained mental health chaplain straddles the world of spirituality and medicine, I am rightly seen as the legitimate person with whom to raise such matters. My presence in the world of spirituality, religious belief and pastoral care, along with my training in mental healthcare, provides me with a unique opportunity to help in the provision of holistic care, alongside the rest of the MDT. As a chaplain, I possess a particular speciality or understanding of the relation between faith, illness and the emotional conflicts that can arise in a person's thinking. My training and experience in the world of spirituality and religious belief perhaps allows me more freedom to be less sceptical of a client's judgements. In this way, I, as chaplain, complement the expertise of the MDT. Working together and establishing strong links across the MDT puts the shared task of working towards the holistic recovery of clients at the top of the agenda.

In psychiatric care, where clients experience a wide range of difficulties – emotional, physical, mental, social and spiritual – care must be given to the client as a whole person, and a chaplain contributes significantly to that holistic care. Spiritual care is a key component of the healing process and, where a client is supported in this aspect of their life, there is more potential benefit for increased well-being. I believe in witches no more than the doctor concerned with Yesuto, but I take seriously the impact that beliefs can have on a person. My openness to the client helped him to feel understood. I held him in a safe space, and that safety allowed him to explore his beliefs and challenge his spiritual and cultural conditioning.

Conclusion

As a chaplain, I am open to all things, all possibilities; the realm of the unknown and the unknowable. I stand in (or represent) the space between this world and the next; hence, I was called upon when religion and witches reared their head in the consultation room. This case study demonstrates how culture and spirituality impact upon people, on their mental health and well-being, and the role that a chaplain may play in this interaction. The study also demonstrates that simply meeting the client at their point of contact, listening respectfully and taking them seriously, and allowing them to discuss their spiritual experience proved to be healing. People's spiritual or religious beliefs should not be interpreted as symptoms of disordered minds. In order for us to function fully, no part of our lives should be denigrated or denied; all aspects of our lives need to be addressed. Focusing on the illness to the detriment of all else is to reduce a person to the level of their illness.

Since it is essentially intangible and subjective, spirituality is different and idiosyncratic for each person (McDonald and Schreyer 1991). Unfortunately, because of this, the 'spiritual life is always in danger of being restricted to higher or, so it is believed, more important areas than those in which most human beings live. But at its best, spirituality concerns the meaning of everyday life' (Carr 1989, p.155). When we start to see spirituality in everything, we can begin to negotiate the crossroads where spirituality, illness and healing meet. Mental illness can be a devastating experience in people's lives, and paying heed to their spirituality can assist and help to sustain them. Ultimately, spirituality can enhance people's lives, encourage healing and alleviate emotional and physical suffering (Wilding, May and Muir-Cochrane 2005). Since spirituality is vitally important for sustaining mental and emotional well-being, an integrative approach to healthcare is crucial. Such a holistic approach means starting conversations about spirituality with clients in the consultation room and having a commitment to learning more about how spirituality impacts on their lives.

References

Agang, S. (2009) 'Who's afraid of witches? Among African Christians, too many of us are.' *Christianity Today*. Available at www.christianitytoday.com/ct/2009/septemberweb-only/137-21.0.html, accessed on 4 July 2014.

Awolalu, J.O. (1975) 'What is African traditional religion?' *Studies in Comparative Religion 9*, 1, 1–28. Available at www.studiesincomparativereligion.com/Public/articles/What_is_African_Traditional_Religion-by_Joseph_Omosade_Awolalu.aspx, accessed on 4 July 2014.

Bannerman-Richter, G. (1982) *The Practice of Witchcraft in Ghana*. Winona, MN: Apollo Books.

Beck, A.T., Rush, A.J., Shaw, B.F. and Emery, G. (1979) *Cognitive Therapy of Depression*. New York, NY: Guildford Press.

Carr, W. (1989) *The Pastor as Theologian*. London: SPCK.

Cox, J. (1996) 'Psychiatry and religion: A general psychiatrist's perspective.' In D. Bhugra (ed) *Psychiatry and Religion: Context, Consensus and Controversy*. London: Routledge, pp.157–166.

Cuéllar, I. and Paniagua, F.A. (2000) *Handbook of Multicultural Mental Health: Assessment and Treatment of Diverse Populations*. London: Academic Press.

Dein, S. (2004) 'Working with patients with religious beliefs.' *Advances in Psychiatric Treatment 10*, 287–294.

Dein, S., Cook, C.C.H., Powell, A. and Eagger, S. (2010) 'Religion, spirituality and mental health.' *The Psychiatrist Online 34*, 63–64. Available at pb.rcpsych.org/content/34/2/63.full, accessed on 4 July 2014.

Ellis, S. and ter Haar, G. (2004) *Worlds of Power: Religious Thought and Political Practice in Africa*. New York, NY: Oxford University Press.

Greenberg, D. and Witztum, E. (1991) 'Problems in the treatment of religious patients.' *American Journal of Psychotherapy 45*, 4, 554–565.

Hick, S.F. and Bien, T. (eds) (2008) *Mindfulness and the Therapeutic Relationship*. New York, NY: Guildford Press.

Kim-Goh, M. (1993) 'Conceptualization of mental illness among Korean-American clergymen and implications for mental health service delivery.' *Community Mental Health Journal 29*, 5, 405–412.

La Fontaine, J. (2012) 'Witchcraft belief is a curse on Africa.' *The Guardian*, 1 March. Available at www.theguardian.com/commentisfree/belief/2012/mar/01/witchcraft-curse-africa-kristy-bamu, accessed on 4 July 2014.

LeDoux, J. (1998) 'Fear and the brain: Where have we been and where are we going?' *Biological Psychiatry 44*, 12, 1229–1238.

Marshall, W.L. and Serran, G.A. (2004) 'The role of the therapist in offender treatment.' *Psychology, Crime & Law 10*, 3, 309–320.

McDonald, B.L. and Schreyer, R. (1991) 'Spiritual benefits of leisure participation and leisure settings.' In B. Driver, P. Brown and G. Peterson (eds) *Benefits of Leisure*. State College, PA: Venture Publishing, 179–194.

Mearns, D. and Thorne, B. (1996) *Person-Centred Counselling in Action*. London: Sage.

Meyer, D. (2011) 'Cognitive Behavioural Theory.' In S. Degges-White and N.L. Davis (eds) *Integrating the Expressive Arts into Counseling Practice: Theory-Based Interventions*. New York, NY: Springer, 45–64.

Nicholls, V. (2002) 'Taken seriously: The Somerset spirituality project.' Available at www.mentalhealth.org.uk/content/assets/PDF/publications/taken-seriously.pdf, accessed on 4 July 2014.

Palmer, K. (2010) *Spellbound: Inside West Africa's Witch Camps*. New York, NY: Free Press.

Pfeifer, S. (1994) 'Belief in demons and exorcism in psychiatric patients in Switzerland.' *British Journal of Medical Psychology 67*, 3, 247–258.

Rogers, C.R. (1980) *A Way of Being*. Boston, MA: Houghton Mifflin.

Rogers, C.R. (1986) 'A client-centered, person-centered approach to therapy.' In L. Kutash and A. Wolf (eds) *Psychotherapist's Casebook: Theory and Technique in the Practice of Modern Therapists*. San Francisco, CA: Jossey-Bass.

Trenholm, P., Trent, J. and Compton, W.C. (1998) 'Negative religious conflict as a predictor of panic disorder.' *Journal of Clinical Psychology 54*, 1, 59–65.

Ukst-Margetic, B. and Margetic, B. (2005) 'Religiosity and health outcomes: Review of literature.' *Collegium Antropologicum 29*, 1, 365–371.

Wagner, M.W. (2006) *Exploring the Therapeutic Relationship: Practical Insights for Today's Clinician*. Sandy, UT: Ecko House.

Wilding, C., May, E. and Muir-Cochrane, E. (2005) 'Experience of spirituality, mental illness and occupation: A life-sustaining phenomenon.' *Australian Occupational Therapy Journal 52*, 1, 2–9.

Winbolt, B. (2011) *Solution Focused Therapy for the Helping Professions*. London: Jessica Kingsley Publishers.

Chapter 7

'I tried to kill myself. Will God keep me apart from the person I love in the life-after?'

— June, a 78-year-old woman who attempted suicide

Christopher Swift

Introduction

This case concerns the spiritual care of June, a 78-year-old woman who was admitted to an acute hospital following a suicide attempt. In addition to health problems associated with the attempt to take her life, the patient had suffered from emphysema for many years. The context for June's encounter with me was a general medical ward of a 450-bed district general hospital on the outskirts of a major city in England. The case is unusual and has been chosen in order to identify and analyse the components of my intervention. While the encounter may not be described as a typical chaplaincy case (if such a thing exists), it is rich in issues that are present in some form across a range of spiritual care interventions. These issues include: mortality; self-harm; ideas of judgement; the chaplain's identity; ethics and integrity; sexuality; ward culture; theology; and perceptions of God.

This case arose 5 years into my ordained ministry and in the second year of my work as a part-time hospital chaplain. I held a joint appointment as an Anglican Team Vicar (4 days a week) and coordinator of a team of part-time chaplains (2 days a week). Funding from the hospital went to the Team, and not directly to me. I held a long-range pager, and in all other respects I appeared to enjoy the same access and involvement as employees of a National Health Service (NHS) hospital; however, as this case demonstrates, the level of integration with other NHS professions was weak.

Despite the division of time noted above, with the hospital less than 2 miles away, the elements of my joint appointment were interspersed on a daily basis. My involvement in chaplaincy at all was the consequence of other life events, particularly the need to relocate at the time I married another minister. Research in England has noted that the move into chaplaincy is often associated with personal circumstances (Hancocks, Sherbourne and Swift 2008). Due to the combined nature of my role, the length of time to train for both functions (new vicar training plus chaplaincy) was protracted. Reflective practice and case study analysis were not required, although opportunities for both arose during residential cell-group meetings (critical peer support), spiritual direction and formal training in counselling skills. I had taken a 4-day introductory course for newly appointed healthcare chaplains provided by the Church of England, funded by the NHS, and was completing an MA in Theology, with a dissertation focusing on ethical issues in intensive care. I was 29 years old.

The case presented here occurred 20 years ago. The patient in question had lost her next-of-kin and there were no other close relationships in her life. While there was no one for me to contact to gain permission to feature aspects of our encounters in this study, I have nevertheless changed her name and the location of the hospital has been anonymized. The material presented below is based on contemporaneous journal notes which accurately reflect the circumstances and language found in each encounter.

Case study

Encounter 1

I received a paged call during normal working hours. The ward relayed the request from a patient to see 'a padre'. Attending the nursing station on the ward within 10 minutes, I was briefed that the patient concerned, June, had attempted to take her own life. She had been found at home following an overdose of pills, and was making a good recovery in hospital. June was 78 years old and suffered from an underlying condition of emphysema. I had not previously met the patient, so a nurse told me more about her.

The nurse soon led me to this patient, who was wearing her own clothes and sitting by a bed.

Nurse: Hello, June. This is the chaplain you asked for. (*June looks up.*)

Chaplain: Hello, June, I'm Chris. I'm a Church of England chaplain here at the hospital.

June: Can we talk somewhere privately? I can get about a bit.

June and I look at the nurse.

Nurse: Yes, I don't see why not. We have a Day Room, and I'll just check it's empty.

The nurse moves a few yards across the ward and through a partly open door.

June: Are you a chaplain or a God-botherer?

I clearly convey some confusion in my facial response to June's question.

June: I was in the Royal Air Force. Whenever new chaplains came to our unit we used to keep an eye on them and work out whether they were interested in evangelizing people or helping people. We called the first lot God-botherers and the second lot chaplains. Word would soon go round about which you were.

At this point the nurse returns.

Nurse: Yes, that'll be fine. There's no one in there at the moment.

The nurse returns to her station. June gets up a little unsteadily and walks across to where the nurse has been. I follow her. There are about a dozen chairs in the room, which appears a bit disorganized. I bring a chair close to the one June is heading towards, the one nearest the door. She sits down with a sigh. At this point, her demeanour changes, and she is less composed than a moment ago.

> *June:* I should be dead. I want to be dead. Those bloody doctors. I played heck with them when they'd brought me round and told me what happened. I was so angry I cried. 'Why didn't you just leave me as I was?' I kept asking. I can't believe what's happened.

> *Chaplain:* Take your time June.

> *June:* I didn't want to upset anyone. The day before I took the pills I sent a letter second class to the local police station. I didn't want anyone to come in and be shocked to find me dead. But the post office delivered it the next day! Can you believe it? So the police came round and found that I was unconscious but still alive. That's when they called an ambulance. (*tearfully*) You see, my partner died a few months ago. We'd been together for years. When she died, well…I've got emphysema. I'll never get it cured, it's just managed. But I'll die soon enough. I thought, 'What's the point of going on?' I just want to be with the person I love. Is that wrong? (*pause*) Listen, I need to ask you something. Because I've tried to kill myself, do you think God will keep me apart from the person I love, you know, in the life-after?

> *Chaplain:* June, I…

> *June:* Don't give me any flannel. I need to know what you really believe. You've got to tell me that, haven't you? What will happen? Will we be kept apart, separated as some kind of punishment?

> *Chaplain:* No. I don't believe that God will punish you because of what you've done. God isn't vindictive. A lot of people believe that the experience of love is the closest we get to God.

June becomes calmer.

> *June:* Nothing's changed. I still wish I were dead. But here I am, stuck in the land of the living. I don't know what happens now. Do you know?

> *Chaplain:* No. I'm sure if you ask the staff they'll tell you.

> *June:* I don't know if I trust them.

> *Chaplain:* Why do you think that June, has something happened?

> *June:* Last night. Last night I heard them giggling about me. I think they'd read something in my notes, maybe the letter I'd written before taking the pills was in there. They seemed to find it funny that someone my age loved another woman as much as I did. (*She is tearful again.*)

> *Chaplain:* That's terrible. Would you like me to speak to a senior nurse about this?

> *June:* No, it'll just make matters worse. I don't know what to think anymore. I just want to be with her!

Encounter 2 (the following day)

> *Chaplain:* Hello, June, how are you doing?

> *June:* Good, I'm glad you've come. Let's go to the Day Room.

We walk the short distance to the Day Room, which is vacant, and sit down near each other. The door remains ajar.

> *Chaplain:* How are you feeling?

> *June:* Alright, I suppose. (*Several moments of silence follow.*) Nothing's changed. (*She becomes tearful and agitated.*) Why couldn't they have just left me? I'm no good to anyone else, there's nothing here for me to live for… (*She is unable to continue for a moment.*) If they'd left me alone, it would all be over now.

Chaplain: I'm sorry, June. I can't imagine what you must be feeling.

June: (*Composing herself.*) It's just that we lived for each other. We didn't have any friends to speak of, hardly knew the neighbours. I've a brother, but we haven't been in touch for years.

Chaplain: When we first met you asked me about God and what had happened. Is faith something that's been important for you?

June: Well, yes and no. I think I told you that I was in the Air Force? Well, going to chapel and church was what you did. There were church parades and things. Some padres were good, others you kept well away from. One arranged for me to be confirmed. After that I went into some churches now and then but never settled anywhere. We weren't sure we'd always be welcome. But I've kept believing, and since she died… (*tearfully*) since she died, and the funeral, maybe it's mattered more. Do you know, on the day she died I left here…I can't imagine the state I was in…and I just drove until I found a church that was open, and I went in and prayed. Now [that] she's gone I have nothing left.

Chaplain: You mentioned being confirmed. Has receiving Communion been something important for you?

June: Well, it was, but it's been years since I last took it.

Chaplain: Might it be something you want to do while in hospital? I could bring you Communion if you would like that?

June: Could you? Yes, yes, I'd like that. It's been a long time, but yes, that would be good.

Encounter 3 (4 days later)

Chaplain: Hello, June.

June: (*Immediately getting up.*) Day Room please. (*She leads the way to our regular meeting place. We enter and sit down.*) I've got a dilemma.

Chaplain: Oh?

June: Yes. I've got to go to some sort of assessment meeting…you know, with psychiatrists or psychologists or something.

Chaplain: Why's that a dilemma?

June: You know what I feel. I want to do this again when I get out. I can't see any reason to go on living and every reason to die. But if I say that, if I tell them how I really feel, they might section me [detain her under mental health laws]. So I've got a choice. Do I lie and get my freedom, or tell them the truth and be kept locked up?

Chaplain: That's quite a problem.

June: What would you do? Do you think I'm being unreasonable?

Chaplain: June, I can't judge what you feel. But I can understand from what you've said about why you feel this way. You've been very honest about your situation and you clearly understand the course your illness is likely to take. There isn't an easy answer to your dilemma. In the time I've known you, I appreciate how much integrity means to you.

June: That's the problem. I feel I'm going to have to lie to get my freedom. I don't like that; I don't like that at all. To sit there and smile and say, 'I've learned my lesson; I won't do it again; it was just a blip'. It stinks! But I don't want to be locked up either. What should I do?

Chaplain: June…I don't know. I appreciate the choice you're facing, but I can't see that there's an easy answer.

June: (*A few moments of silence pass.*) Would you be there?

Chaplain: Where?

June: Would you come to support me at the meeting? They said I could bring someone with me, but there isn't anyone. Would you come? I'm not asking you to say anything, just to be there. I'd find it helpful to have you there with me. Would you do that?

Chaplain: If I can, I will. When you have a date and time let me know. Of course I'll come to support you.

Other encounters

Not all my encounters with June are recorded above. I took her Holy Communion during one of my visits. In a simple and quiet service, once again in the under-occupied Day Room, June was tearful and largely silent. In the prayers, I asked that as June's partner was now close to God, we would know God to be close to us. The reading I chose was from 1 Corinthians 13, a few verses from the great exaltation of love. It felt to me that love was the most positive quality June had spoken about – a point of connection between Scripture and her experience. After the 10-minute service, June simply said, 'Thank you.'

June's admission to hospital lasted 2 weeks. I continued to support June during her stay, visiting once every 2 or 3 days. We only shared Communion on one occasion, although she requested that I make contact with her local church in order to continue this when she returned home. I attended the meeting June had with the psychiatric assessment team. I witnessed June telling the panel that she had made a mistake; she understood the error of her ways; it would not happen again. June was believed and discharged soon afterwards. I don't know that her words alone, and my silent complicity with them, influenced the decision for her to be discharged. It was part of a package of information and evidence, including her local doctor's input and ward observations, which the panel assessed. But I cannot avoid the question of how I would have felt if June had left the hospital and immediately taken her life. Her physical state had stabilized, and it was decided that she was well enough to return home without any intermediate care. June's general practitioner would be advised of her hospital stay and its outcome, but I do not know what ongoing care that may have resulted in.

In my final visit to June in hospital I noted how she had changed. I did not know whether she would leave hospital and take an overdose the next day. The pain of bereavement still overshadowed her, but the anger had diminished. During the early visits, June only spoke of the time since her partner's death and her own fury at being revived by the medics. Now the prompt delivery of her letter to the police was described with a wry sense of irony. Circumstances seemed to be telling June 'not yet'.

Before June left she thanked me, and I decided to tell her that, if she needed to, I could be contacted by the hospital switchboard. This is not something I did in all circumstances, and perhaps a bit of me was anxious that June might return to the state of mind that had led to her suicide attempt. I didn't want to shut the door on a pastoral relationship June had found useful, even though at June's request I had arranged a hand-over to a local cleric, as she wished to continue receiving Communion.

My final contact with June took place a year and a half later, on Christmas Day. I was called around lunchtime by a nurse on the intensive care unit (ICU) of a hospital a few miles from the one where I worked. June had apparently asked for me to be called, although she had since lost consciousness and was not expected to survive the day. I decided to attend the hospital and found June in precisely those circumstances she had so much wanted to avoid at the end of her life. Various tubes were in her body; sensors were attached and oxygen was being delivered at high volume. I spoke to June, but there was no response. I sat for several minutes by June's bed, addressed by the situation she was in. It felt a little as though this was a lesson for me, and a vindication of June's determination to die peacefully in her own bed surrounded by pictures of her partner and the comfort of familiar things. After sitting by her, I stood and informed the nurse that I was going to say some prayers for June. I spoke to June, explaining what I was about to do, and recited the familiar words of an old man at the end of his life, seeing the completion of things and commending himself to God (Luke 2: 29–32). I said the Lord's Prayer, which in some form or another is common to all Christians and feels to me like a thread connecting those key moments in life all the way from baptism to death. Finally, I said the blessing of Aaron (Numbers 6: 24–26) and marked June's forehead with the sign of the cross, repeating the moment when she was baptized – mindful of that other birth about to take place. June seemed peaceful and impassive throughout the prayers.

The machines laboured with regularity beside her. Before going, I asked the nurse to phone me when she died, then I left. The call came within an hour of my return home.

Discussion

For various reasons the case was significant for me, and I have used aspects of the situation in subsequent chaplaincy training. While several decades have passed, the issues it raises are still pertinent, and the passage of time perhaps enables me to be more critical in my reflection on the case than I might be with something more immediate. I hope this questioning of my own role is frank and helpful, and useful in emphasizing the importance of reflective practice and thorough preparation for chaplaincy work. There is at least one aspect of the case where I regret not engaging in a more active response to information.

Throughout our conversations, I didn't challenge June about the attempt to take her life. I am not sure where it came from (training or experience, or both), but I was aware of a temptation to go prospecting. It is something I had observed in other staff with patients who expressed a desire to die. The person with the patient is so uncomfortable with the idea that someone might have a good reason to die that they dig about, with increasing anxiety, to present the patient with a nugget of life they feel they should want to live for. 'Have you got grandchildren? Do you like going on holiday? Are you getting ready for Christmas?' Whether what the patient says is truly meant or not, what is wanted most of all is to have feelings heard and acknowledged. The advice to medical practitioners is no less relevant to chaplains: 'any moralizing attitude should be avoided, using careful and exploratory evaluative listening of the issues and personal motivations of the subject' (Boloş, Ciubară and Chiriță 2013, p.77).

The identity of the chaplain as someone often in the company of the dying may lend an added significance to the recognition of a wish to die. To take June's feelings seriously is an act which affirms her dignity.

By being open to her situation June makes a rational case that there is no further point in continuing to live. Despite the length of time which has elapsed, June's situation remains pastorally relevant, and politically significant, in the context of repeated attempts in the UK to pass legislation for a 'right to die'.

Assessment and interventions

The assessment of religious and spiritual need is a dynamic process. In the case study, the limited information given over the phone from the ward was amplified by the encounter with the patient. As the episode of care developed, various themes emerged, some directly and others less obviously. I was conscious from the start that June was evaluating me even as I was assessing her needs, and the relationship of care would be shaped by the success of establishing an effective connection in a short space of time. At the stage in my career in chaplaincy when the case arose, I did not use a formal assessment tool, but based my analysis of the situation on pastoral care training. This drew on a form of the pastoral cycle (Poling 1984), focusing on the interplay of action, reflection, analysis and new action.

During our first encounter, I was quickly made aware of June's spiritual and religious needs. The nature of the initial request had indicated a familiarity with the role of a chaplain, and June appeared to have a clear sense of what she wanted. The introduction I made to June noted my denominational identity. This may have been helpful in that it told June something about my religious formation; but it may have been unhelpful in that it emphasized the religious nature of my role. This is often a tussle for chaplains, balancing openness with a wish to be available for those without a formal faith adherence. It could be that I was responding in part to June's use of the word 'padre', although that could apply to another Christian denomination. It is not always the way I introduce myself today, focusing on my identity as a chaplain first and judging how relevant further information is as the pastoral role develops. The longer I am a chaplain, the less I tend to say.

Even with limited training as a chaplain, I was mindful of the care needed in protecting both the patient and myself in a pastoral encounter in an area out of direct sight from the nursing station: I left the door ajar. Planning ongoing care after my first visit, I identified pastoral support as a key requirement, because the patient was isolated and appeared to have found me to be helpful.

The directness of June's question about the life-after presented a number of possible motives. It could be that her relationship with a same-sex partner, across a lifetime when such arrangements were not socially acceptable, carried with it a sense of disapproval. The linking of Christianity with a condemnation of homosexuality is both an historic and contemporary phenomenon. A similar observation could be made with regard to suicide, and the two factors combined may have stirred in June ideas of a God who might punish her. The question which crystallized was about the nature of God and God's relationship with a person when life is over. Would God punish June by preventing the outcome which her failed suicide attempt was intended to achieve – that she and the person she loved would be together?

From the perspective of spiritual care, June manifested several areas for consideration and concern:

- recent bereavement

- a desire to end her bereavement through her own death

- theological anxiety about the nature of God in relation to moral issues

- acute isolation

- a tentative connection with church life and sacraments.

Aspects of June's character revealed in this first encounter appealed to me. June was plain spoken, able to articulate her feelings and needs, and was sensitive to irony, even in the midst of traumatic and testing personal experiences. A care for others was demonstrated in her arrangement for the police to discover her body. June was also the victim of prejudice and casual cruelty. It was not difficult for me to like June, and respect her honesty and directness. The experiences she had faced, and the future she imagined, are consistent with the personal challenges faced by many in the elderly population (MacKinley 2012).

In responding to June's need, I allowed time and engaged in attentive listening (Mundle and Smith 2013). Theological concerns were weighed against pastoral priorities, and what I said was carefully considered in order not to inflame the situation or cause further isolation or feelings of rejection. The attention of the chaplain in these circumstances constitutes bridge building to the patient's experience, and it enabled June to share intimate and distressful thoughts about her life. My role also absorbed some of the anger directed by June at the hospital staff, who were, in her view, guilty of acting against her wishes. It is not unusual for strong emotions to emerge in this kind of situation (Coghlan and Ali 2009).

A question worth considering in this case is whether June was, consciously or unconsciously, manipulating me. June had found someone she believed she could tell about her life and about her persisting wish to commit suicide. At the same time, implicitly, June assumed that I would not share these views with other hospital staff. This is a unique risk for hospital chaplains, when patients may have a general view that anything shared with a priest is sacrosanct. In this case, I should have found a suitable moment to explain to June my responsibilities, both professionally and within the NHS. This is not an easy call in any situation, especially where such a formal explanation risks breaking a pastoral relationship which is just emerging. If anything, it suggests that part-time chaplaincy staff, including volunteers, need at least as much (if not more) training in this regard than their full-time colleagues.

This aspect of the case highlights the deficiency of interprofessional cooperation. I did not discuss the situation at the time with a psychiatrist at the hospital or a senior nurse on the ward. When I accompanied June to a meeting with psychiatrists I was there as a supporter for June, rather than part of her multidisciplinary care team. I could not be certain that June was lying about her understanding of what had happened and what she intended to do in the future. There was a risk that June would make a fresh attempt on her life. From the perspective of hospital regulations for staff conduct, as well as the obligations of collegial working, a case could be made that I had acted unwisely. The UK Board of Healthcare Chaplaincy (UKBHC) *Code of Conduct for Healthcare Chaplains* (2014b) for healthcare chaplains states an intention to promote 'the well being of those in their care' (1.1). This in itself raises fundamental questions about human well-being in the context of ethics and theology. Does the continuation of physical life at all costs promote the well-being of the person? The chaplain in this situation has obligations to both protect the vulnerable and act to safeguard the interests of the patient. In supporting June, I tacitly agreed that she was competent to make reasonable decisions, even while experiencing acute bereavement. I arrived at this conclusion based on my personal judgment without the use of any formal assessment or algorithm. In retrospect, I realize that it would have been helpful to check my perceptions about June's integrity and logical thinking with other members of the care team. One way to approach this would have been to find another chaplain – one working in elderly mental health – to discuss the situation and receive more experienced advice. Reviewing the original case, I can see that my choice not to alert others to what June had shared created a potential risk. Given June's actions in preparing for the discovery of her body, I didn't believe that she presented any risk to others; however, she remained a risk to her own physical well-being. Had I represented the concerns she confided in me to others, June might have received some prioritized bereavement support or treatment which would have diminished her suicidal intentions. Equally, she may have been detained in a psychiatric unit until she persuaded clinical staff that her conversations with me had been misguided. Ethically, I placed a high value on June's autonomy, but less on whether my inaction would expose her to harm. I did not disagree with June's analysis of her situation or the understanding she held about her medical prognosis. Life for her was not going to be good – nor was it going to be very long. The key role of my intervention in June's care was the sober and sincere acknowledgement of her situation, done by someone of perceived neutrality whose identity and ritual practice linked this world and the next. Only a chaplain could fulfil this role for June.

June's case is unusual in that it presented an explicit and coherent theological concern. It also generated a situation where the ambiguous identity of the chaplain, as a separate figure within the community (Swift 2009), enabled June to confide in someone she perceived to stand apart from the clinical team. People who practise their faith are a minority in the population, and several studies have noted the challenge staff experience in assessing religion and spirituality (Swift, Calcuttawala and Eliot 2007; Howard *et al.* 2013). Nevertheless, extensive post-discharge patient surveys (which exclude some groups where religious needs may be more pronounced, such as the dying) continue to register over 17% of patients who say that they wish to practice their religion while in hospital (Clayton 2012). Certainly June believed that the person with the knowledge and skill to respond to her challenging situation was the padre.

Outcomes

At the time this case took place, chaplaincy in the UK was even less concerned with defined outcomes than it is today. The rising economic pressures in healthcare, as well as the simple fact that it would be good to know what helps or hinders patients, have led researchers to call for more attention to be paid to outcomes (Cadge 2012).

The most successful element of the spiritual care provided for June lay in the pastoral relationship she was able to establish with the chaplain, coupled with a reconnection to the Christian sacrament of the Eucharist. The ability to form a relationship with the patient, quickly and effectively, is a primary skill for the healthcare chaplain. In some situations a previous history of chaplaincy care allows a trusting relationship to develop at surprising speed (equally, there are, of course, circumstances where that history may be a barrier to the encounter).

There are two aspects of the outcomes where spiritual care failed to achieve what June wanted: first, that she was somehow dissuaded, whether by conscious decision or want of opportunity, from subsequent attempts on her life; second, that she eventually had the kind of death she so desperately wished to avoid. For June, these two issues were inextricably linked. Had the 'right to die' existed in the UK at the time of June's hospital admission, her situation may have developed very differently.

There is insufficient information available to know whether more could have been done to support June in her final illness. Hospice care may have enabled a more dignified and less clinical experience in the final days of her life. While a referral was made for June to continue to receive spiritual support in the community, this inevitably marks a letting go of involvement with a patient. Since June's death, care at the end of life in the UK has received more attention,[1] and there is an intention to discuss with patients, while still relatively well, how they would like to be cared for in their final days. At the same time, efforts to emulate the perceived excellence of the hospice setting in acute care have become a matter of public concern (Hawkes 2013). In June's case, without someone to advocate for her concerns, the medical profession acted to preserve and sustain her physical life; however, even today, it cannot be ruled out that sudden illness would mean a patient in June's situation still ends up in intensive care.

June's calculated attempt to control the ending of her life failed due to an unexpected event in the process: the letter to the police arriving earlier than anticipated. Without any official mechanism to achieve what she desired, and perhaps believing it to be in her best interests, June had no option other than to concoct a home-made plan. Inevitably, this meant she could not risk telling anyone before it took place.

There are several risks in presenting a case such as this. I am in the middle of it as both actor and author. I cannot separate myself from it, and there is an inevitable tendency to tell the tale in ways that influence the reader. There are several points in the situation where I would now act differently. The case itself contributed to my appreciation of alternative actions, as have many more years of pastoral practice and greater involvement in reflective work and chaplaincy education. In particular:

- I would have sought advice from a senior nurse in the hospital about what might be done to act in some way on June's comments about being mocked by night staff. June may not have wished me to act on this, but the organization could have responded in some way to remind staff about their behaviour. The Francis Report in England has highlighted the lack of dignity given to patients and the need for change in nursing practice (Hayter 2013). Pastoral care must extend beyond the personal and engage the political, if it is to be meaningful.

- A part-time chaplain in particular can often feel like an outsider in the hospital. Chaplaincy care in these circumstances can seem more like an incursion than a fully included element of the multidisciplinary team. There is no easy answer to this, but it is unlikely that others will strive to include the chaplain unless the chaplain makes a determined effort to be involved. Difficult as it is, a way must be found for this to be done, especially in places of care without any full-time presence.

In hospital, June saw little before her other than a progressive decline in health, alone and culminating in death – possibly in the sterile and high-tech environment of an ICU. Given the context for June's death, I cannot avoid the feeling that, in some small way, my involvement and subsequent church contact helped steer her away from a further attempt on her life. Yet, between hospital and community spiritual care support, had we failed in helping June die with the dignity and peace she wanted?

I believe that, in our encounters, I witnessed a reawakening of spiritual awareness in June. I am conscious now, looking back, that patients can sometimes latch on to a member of staff and invest them with a saviour role. In that light, I can see the risk that June's interest in Holy Communion may have arisen from a desire to please me – to engage with something she knew I would value. That may have been an aspect of what took place, but I do not believe it was the whole story. In her state of devastation after her partner's death, our meetings and Holy Communion appear to have provided some tentative underpinning to her existence. In responding to the complexity of June's concerns, both pastoral affirmation and ritual participation appear to have been important. While I cannot know precisely what June's participation in Communion meant for her, it is recognized that such a service embodies powerful themes of relationship (Green 1985). These themes include connection to the church (in this world and the next), connection to God and connection to a personal history, including childhood. It is helpful that the liturgy of Holy Communion is largely prescribed, making links without labouring the detail of previous pastoral encounters. But it is all there: confession, forgiveness, thanksgiving, love, betrayal and a body broken and shared. Relationships could still be formed, and the image of a punitive God could give way to one of acceptance and reconciliation.

Conclusion

From the outset June had shown a concern for integrity and openness. This was confirmed by her subsequent anxiety about her intention to try to end her life. Without any significant person left alive for her, and in the context of a debilitating and deteriorating physical condition, June presented her determination to attempt suicide again as a rational and reasonable choice. June realized that to say so risked forced detention under mental health legislation. She neither wished to lie nor lose her freedom. As the chaplain, I was placed in an uneasy position between religious teaching about the sacredness of life and pastoral care of June;

however, I did not believe that June's thinking was uninformed or unreasonable, although it was undoubtedly shaped by the experience of grief.

This case study touches on some profound issues about the purpose of life and the prospect of death. As the longevity of people in the West continues to increase, it is more likely that people will experience the loss of their partners at an advanced age. Facing such a traumatic event at any time of life is difficult, but when age suggests there are only a few years of life left, it can become difficult to move through immediate bereavement and find fresh purpose in life. Since caring for June I have had similar cases, and what I learned through this first experience has helped inform the later interventions. As a full-time chaplain, I feel more integrated into the multidisciplinary team and find that other staff face the same dilemmas and concerns I experienced; however, there continues to be a sense of ambiguity around the role of the chaplain for some staff, and considerable variation in the extent to which chaplains are included in care teams in the UK.

Many years after this case study, I served as President of the UK's College of Health Care Chaplains. During my time in office, I addressed meetings across the country and was asked on several occasions about our work towards creating a formal register of professional chaplains. Part-time chaplains in particular were concerned about any further requirements for training and ongoing reflection. Unlike chaplaincies in countries such as the USA, being a chaplain in England did not (and still does not) require a common route of entry to the profession. Work is taking place to clarify this, but the reality remains that chaplains are permitted significant latitude in their practice. Both the NHS and the UKBHC have produced guidance about chaplaincy competencies (UKBHC 2014a) and a Code of Conduct is maintained by the professional bodies (UKBHC 2014b).

Understandably, part-time chaplains struggle to see how the demands of parish life and the need to meet professional requirements in the NHS could be balanced; however, the case I have described illustrates the difficulty in having two or even three tiers of capability for chaplaincy practice. While distinctions for planned work can be made (such as training, research and projects), any chaplain participating in an on-call service can face the most complex scenarios from day one. In many cases, back-up advice can be obtained from a more experienced colleague, but such need may not be recognized until the pastoral encounter is well underway. Establishing thorough training for part-time chaplains can be difficult, but thorough training is essential for any chaplain participating in an urgent-response service. In the UK this work is progressing, albeit slowly. In other countries Clinical Pastoral Education provides a coherent path of formation, with commonly recognized levels of attainment. It is also a path which encourages the use of case studies for reflective practice (Schipani 2012). Chaplains cannot be shy about the difference excellent spiritual and religious care can make to patients' lives.

Endnote

1   See www.dyingmatters.org.

References

Boloş, A., Ciubară, A. and Chiriţă, R. (2013) 'Moral and ethical aspects of the relationship between depression and suicide.' *Revista Romana de Bioetica 10*, 3, 71–79.

Cadge, W. (2012) *Paging God: Religion in the Halls of Medicine.* Chicago, IL: The Chicago University Press.

Clayton, A. (2012) 'Unpicking the religious profile of NHS inpatient populations.' *The Journal of Health Care Chaplaincy 12*, 1, 65–76.

Coghlan, C. and Ali, I. (2009) 'Suicide.' In C. Cook, A. Powell and A. Sims (eds) *Spirituality and Psychiatry.* London: The Royal College of Psychiatrists, 61–80.

Green, R. (1985) *Only Connect.* London: Darton Longman and Todd.

Hancocks, G., Sherbourne, J. and Swift, C. (2008) '"Are they refugees?" Why Church of England male clergy enter healthcare chaplaincy.' *Practical Theology 1*, 2, 163–179.

Hawkes, N. (2013) 'Liverpool care pathway is scrapped after review finds it was not well used.' *British Medical Journal 347.*

Hayter, M. (2013) 'The UK Francis Report: The key messages for nursing.' *Journal of Advanced Nursing 69*, 8, 1–3.

Howard, N., Snowdon, A., Telfer, I. and Waller, R. (2013) 'Recognizing and meeting the spiritual needs of hospital inpatients.' *Health & Social Care Chaplaincy 1*, 1, 35–48.

MacKinlay, E. (2012) *Palliative Care, Ageing and Spirituality: A Guide for Older People, Carers and Families.* London, UK: Jessica Kingsley Publishers.

Mundle, R. and Smith, B. (2013) 'Hospital chaplains and embodied listening: Engaging with stories and the body in healthcare environments.' *Illness, Crisis & Loss 21*, 2, 95–108.

Poling, J.N. (1984) 'Ethical reflection and pastoral care, part I.' *Pastoral Psychology 32*, 2, 106–114.

Schipani, D.S. (2012) 'Case study method.' In B. Miller-McLemore (ed) *The Wiley-Blackwell Companion to Practical Theology.* Chichester, UK: John Wiley and Sons, 91–101.

Swift, C. (2009) *Hospital Chaplaincy in the Twenty-first Century: The Crisis of Spiritual Care on the NHS.* Farnham, VT: Ashgate Publishing.

Swift, C., Calcuttawala, S. and Eliot, R. (2007) 'Nursing attitudes to recording religious data.' *The British Journal of Nursing 16*, 20, 1279–1282.

UK Board of Healthcare Chaplaincy (UKBHC) (2014a) *Spiritual and Religious Care Capabilities and Competences for Healthcare Chaplains.* Levels 5 and 6. Available at www.ahpcc.org.uk, accessed on 9 January 2015.

UK Board of Healthcare Chaplaincy (UKBHC) (2014b) *Code of Conduct for Healthcare Chaplains.* Available at www.ahpcc.org.uk, accessed on 9 January 2015.

Chapter 8

'My family wants me to see a priest. It can't hurt, right?'

– Nate, a 20-year-old man and his sexual identity

Angelika A. Zollfrank

Introduction

This case study describes my interventions with Nate, a 20-year-old man from the Dominican Republic, admitted to an inpatient medical psychiatric unit after medical treatment subsequent to a serious suicide attempt. As a member of the interdisciplinary team, my goal is to support the treatment, to help the patient's hopefulness and future orientation, as well as to assess and nurture any religious/spiritual coping skills. The distinction between religious behavior, congruent with a religious group, versus support of the patient's dormant personal spirituality, becomes important. This young man struggled in age-appropriate ways with the psychosocial task of identity development and individuation from his family and culture of origin. My interventions were aimed at support of this patient's identity, assistance with religious/spiritual struggle, education in religious/spiritual issues, as well as awareness of religious autonomy. To protect the patient's privacy, key identifiers and circumstances of the case have been altered.

At its heart, this case struggles with an ethical dilemma. Nate's religious struggle and tenuous mental health suggested that he could benefit from being helped to engage with alternative ways of constructing a religious/spiritual orientation that might hold the possibility of positive religious/spiritual coping for him. In this approach the focus would be on empowering Nate to make his own autonomous, adult choices regarding his religious practices and sexual identity. However, Nate came from a cultural background that demanded that choices in support of the values of the community be given priority over choices for individual satisfaction and happiness. Nate was returning to his family, cultural and religious communities, and their value orientation.

A few days before Christmas, Nate was admitted to the emergency department of a large, urban, academic medical center after overdosing on 32.5 grams of APAP (acetaminophen) and 10 grams of NSAID (ibuprofen). Nate had expected to die immediately. When he did not, he sought help, knowing that his suicide attempt had failed. He was brought to the hospital about an hour after the attempt. He was accompanied by his mother's cousin. Nate was born and raised in the Dominican Republic, where his mother still resided. He came to the United States in 2009, and since had lived with his mother's cousin.

In conversation with his psychiatrists, Nate stated that he was not scared by what he had done, and that 'everything in his life had been terrible'. He could not think of anything good. Nate's affect was flat. He was nervous, fidgety and initially cavalier about the suicide attempt, the major impetus for which was his conflict around his sexual orientation. He reported that there was significant longevity in his family, and that he 'could not imagine living another 60 years of a fake life'. Nate refused to speak about his sexual orientation, indicating his shame and guilt; instead, he typed on his cell phone 'gay'. Even embracing his homosexuality internally felt unacceptable to him, and he stated that he was only 'a little bit like that'. He had only confided in his sister, who lived in South Carolina. He felt that if anyone else found out, both he and his family would be ostracized. Such rejection in the community of immigrants from the Dominican Republic would, in effect, be like death for him and his family. While he did not like his father, he did not want his father to have to deal with what Nate believed would be the shame of having a homosexual son. He was very concerned about confidentiality.

Nate had had two prior self-aborted suicide attempts the year before: one through hanging (he had the rope around his neck but did not jump off the support) and one through cutting (as he was about to cut himself, he became fearful of the pain). Since the stressor was chronic, Nate's attempts were very worrisome. The goals of the inpatient stay were to rule out psychosis and major depressive disorder, as well as to help Nate develop new coping strategies. Several routine personality tests were performed: the Wechsler Abbreviated Scale of Intelligence (WASI) (Wechsler 1955); the Personality Assessment Inventory (PAI) (Morey 2007); and the Thematic Apperception Test (TAT) (Aronow, Altman Weiss and Reznikoff 2001). While generally reliable, issues of acculturation, education and verbal skills have been shown to influence the test results, particularly in the WASI (Razani *et al.* 2006). Since Nate's first language was Spanish, and he was under significant stress, test results were referred to with some caution. The patient had no significant medical or psychiatric history and was admitted in the setting of life, religious and social stress. In the United States, suicide is the third leading cause of death for persons between the ages of 15 and 24 years, and it is a very significant, potentially preventable public health issue. Major depressive disorder, anxiety disorders and attempted suicide are highly associated with suicide (Khan *et al.* 2002; Angst, Angst and Strassen 1999). The team's approach was to help Nate imagine that he might be able to cope with and live his identity in the future. This approach was guided by the fact that Nate's conflict had become life-threatening and chronic for him.

Chaplaincy works closely with the interdisciplinary team. The chaplaincy interventions described in this case study took place in the hospital's inpatient medical psychiatric unit. (Details of the case have been discussed with Nate's doctor, who is also the medical director of the unit and who offered invaluable advice about disguising Nate's identity.) The unit is a 24-bed locked adult unit that has the capability to provide medical care as needed. Nate was initially in a private room, as he required intensive psychiatric and ongoing medical supervision. He was then in a semi-private room. Upon admission to the unit a spiritual screening is performed by nursing. Patients are asked their religious and spirituality self-identification and are offered support for any specific religious or spiritual needs or practices during hospitalization. Patients are also asked whether their religious/spiritual practices conflict with medical treatment and whether they would like a visit by a chaplain. Patients' average length of stay is between 8 and 10 days.

I have served the inpatient psychiatric unit for 8 years. I am a Lutheran pastor, a board certified chaplain (Association of Professional Chaplains) and a certified supervisor with the Association for Clinical Pastoral Education. I am a white woman in my forties, with 16 years of ministry experience in the congregation and in the hospital setting. My chaplaincy work in the United States has been exclusively in major academic medical centers. I share with Nate the experience of immigration. He immigrated in 2009 from the Dominican Republic, and I immigrated from Germany 13 years ago. I bring to this encounter the experience of renegotiating my identity in a context different from my culture and family of origin. I have empathy with the considerable stressors of acculturation. Both Nate and I are bilingual. While I consider myself as bicultural and acknowledge losses and gains of life in each culture, Nate is in the *process* of becoming bicultural. I have an 'adopted' family of friends and loved ones in the United States and in Germany. My family of origin resides in Germany. Nate has family in the United States and in the Dominican Republic. Our differences in age, gender, sexual orientation, as well as socioeconomic, denominational and cultural background are significant. During our encounter, I was aware of needing to negotiate these differences.

Case study

Encounter on the day of transfer
to the psychiatric unit

On Nate's first day on the inpatient psychiatric unit, I responded to a request for a Bible. Of note, when patients are transferred from a medical unit to the psychiatric unit, the paper chart is emptied and the process of arriving on the unit equals a new admission. A brief chart review oriented me to his situation. Nate was in the intensive care unit part of the psychiatric unit.

In our brief interaction, Nate was pleasant but did not engage in an extensive conversation. I stated that my purpose for the visit was to bring the Bible he had requested. Nate responded that he had done no such thing – his family had likely asked for the Bible. I apologized and stated that I had no knowledge of the origin of the request, and that I was not there to impose anything on him. I would take the Bible with me again. With flat affect, Nate asked me to leave the Bible on the desk several feet away from his bed, stating it 'wouldn't hurt'. Normalizing a range of religious/ spiritual engagement, I mentioned that some patients found religion or spirituality helpful and others actually felt it to be a source of struggle. What kind of a person was he? In response, Nate stated that he needed to rest. He consented to my offer to come by another day. My chart note stated that Nate was Roman Catholic and had complied with his family's request to have a Bible in his room. I would follow-up as needed.

One of my values is respect for the conflicts, inner turmoil and vulnerability which can leave psychiatric patients confused, overstimulated and aware of their inability to feel, behave or think in ways that are considered 'normal'. Respect can be demonstrated by staying away when patients need to rest in a safe place. From the nurse, I learned more about Nate's family, religious and cultural conflict related to his sexual orientation. The team was very concerned for Nate in his vulnerable state: 'He can't even say the word "gay", he is so terrified.' Staff were intent on creating a safe and healing environment. They safeguarded his right to privacy when his family repeatedly challenged the boundaries of confidentiality. They worked hard to help Nate identify different coping strategies. Psychiatric assessment led to a diagnosis of general anxiety disorder and likely major depressive disorder, which may or may not have been caused by the conflict between Nate's blossoming psychosexual identity and the values of his family, culture and religion. In attempts to support him, it was important to remain attentive to Nate's conflict, rather than trying to resolve it prematurely.

Encounter while rounding

I met Nate again a few days later while rounding. By then Nate had consented to hospitalization and could leave the unit with a 3-day notice. He was sitting in bed, eating and watching television. My goal was to build trust. Nate seemed guarded, uneasy, nervous, wary and suspicious. With highly anxious patients I have learned to carefully observe affect and behavior. I asked Nate about his current emotional state and also about school and plans for the future. He reassured me with a smile that he was feeling much better. This seemed true yet also overemphasized, as if for my sake. He spoke vaguely about applying to different colleges. I was deliberate about not bringing up religious or spiritual topics. My goal was to help Nate feel at ease with me, a chaplain, a religious professional and a representative of teachings that had caused him conflict, fear, isolation and sadness. Dressed in business attire and without clerical collar, I worked towards this goal by attempting to build a relationship with him.

Physical signs of fear and conflict intensified when Nate nervously talked about his family, who were 'so different' from him, wanted him to 'be like them' and 'did not understand him'. He was ruminative, vague and fidgety. Without betraying my knowledge of his sexual identity, I named the conflict in a non-threatening way: 'Your family cares about you but doesn't seem to understand and accept you the way you wish they would.' To counteract his sense of isolation, I normalized and generalized as age appropriate Nate's struggle with his difference in values in relationship to his parents' generation. This led to his talking about the difficulties and hopes related to separating from family and culture of origin in an attempt to establish a meaningful and authentic life.

Nate introduced into our conversation plans of moving out of his mother's cousin's residence, demonstrating some consideration of his future; however, while imagining a different life, he also became more nervous and unable to sustain eye contact. I introduced the idea that in the future he might look back on this current struggle with a greater sense of peace. Nate seemed to find a moment of peace and pleasure in my holding out this hope for him. I was also careful not to press him to talk about his current conflict; however, I did invite, encourage and affirm his hopes, and he shared his dream of applying to law school. This conversation was key to establishing trust. I communicated genuine interest and compassion while not pushing any specific agenda. Nate did not mention his suicide attempt, or the reasons for it, and neither did I. By the end of our conversation, he appeared more open and engaged.

A hallway encounter

On the day of Nate's discharge, we met in the hallway and he requested a Roman Catholic priest. Following our department's procedure, I inquired about the specific sacramental need, and Nate replied that he did not feel he needed a priest, but that his family had requested he go to confession. I proposed that we meet one-on-one to talk more, and he was amenable. Prior to meeting with him, I sought the input of the attending nurse – a liaison between patients, attending physicians, social work and case management. I shared with her that the request was not the patient's request but his family's request. The attending nurse restated the team's goal of empowering Nate to make his own choices and concurred with my plan to support Nate's responsibility and capacity for decision making in religious and spiritual matters as well.

However, I was faced with an ethical dilemma. On the one hand, Nate's religious struggle had become life-threatening to him. He could not see how he could continue living. The value of life is a core ethical value in Nate's Roman Catholic tradition. Based on the ethical principles of vitalism and beneficence, it seemed justifiable to attempt to engage alternative ways of constructing a meaningful religious/spiritual orientation that might hold the possibility for Nate of positive religious/spiritual coping with his sexual identity. In this approach, the focus was on empowering Nate to make autonomous, age-appropriate choices regarding his religious practices and sexual identity. On the other hand, Nate came from a cultural background that valued community and demanded that choices prioritized the values of the community over choices for individual satisfaction and happiness. Nate was returning to his family, cultural and religious communities, and their value orientation. Were the same interventions that aimed at resolution of Nate's conflicts deepening the crisis in which he found himself? In an overly individualistic approach, Nate might lose vital relationships that might increase isolation. With these thoughts in mind, the following conversation took place in a private consultation room.

> *Nate:* (*nervously*) Yes, I thought it would be OK to see a Roman Catholic priest.

> *Chaplain:* (*calmly*) So, tell me again, you said you have a sacramental need?

> *Nate:* (*Embarrassed, fidgety, unsteady eye contact.*) Yes, I want to do the confession-absolution thing. You know, I think it might be a good idea before I leave here.

> *Chaplain:* So, you feel like it would be a good idea to go to confession.

> *Nate:* (*nervously*) Well, it is really more my family who wants me to see a priest. I mean, I am OK going along with it. My aunt [his mother's cousin] wants me to see a priest before I leave. I mean, it can't hurt, right?

> *Chaplain:* Well, I am happy to call a Roman Catholic priest, if this is *your* request. (*Pause, then calmly.*) But I don't think it's a good idea if I call a priest because your family wants you to see a priest. You see, it is your choice, your religious autonomy we are talking about. If *you* want to see a priest, I will call a priest, and he will come up in about

20 minutes. But if it is your *family's* request and not yours, then I am not sure it is honest and a good thing to do.

Nate: (*pensively*) Well, it can't hurt, can it? I mean, I'll just go with it. They seem to be adamant, and I don't really care.

Chaplain: It sounds like you feel some pressure from your family. Is this true?

Nate: Well, yeah…but I'm OK with going with what they want.

Chaplain: I think your problem is that you do not know what to say to your family, if you do not see a priest. Is that true?

Nate: (*Smiling in recognition and with a spark in his eyes.*) Well, yes, that's just it.

Chaplain: I tell you what…how about you tell them that you had a conversation with the chaplain on the unit, who is an ordained pastor of the Lutheran Church. You could say that you got to talk about everything that needed to be talked about, that the conversation took about 45 minutes and that it was meaningful to you.

Nate: (*surprised*) You are a real pastor?

Chaplain: Yes, Masters of Divinity; ordination; the whole nine yards!

Nate: (*smiling*) Sounds like a plan…I mean, I don't feel like I need a priest. *They* just want me to do that.

Chaplain: Yes, you are in a bit of a conflict here. And, correct me if I am wrong, but it doesn't sound like *you* really think you need confession. Is that right?

Nate: (*Looking down.*) Yeah.

Chaplain: So, how about we talk and make it a conversation that is meaningful to you.

Nate: OK. (*smiling*) That sounds good. (*Pause, then with a firmer voice, looking at me.*) I guess I am just really different from my family.

Nate reported that he was looking forward to a time when he would no longer be living with his family, and no longer needed to be 'fake'. He didn't know what to say when relatives pressed him about his romantic life. He didn't date girls and did not want to get married. But his family thought he was at an age where this should be his goal. He stated that he 'didn't like girls that much'. I responded with some education about human sexuality.

> *Chaplain:* This is how I think about it. Human sexuality is a continuum. Some people are clearly heterosexual, and they like to engage with the opposite sex. And then there are people who are very clear that they are attracted to persons of their own sex. And then there are those who are in between these two poles.

> *Nate:* (*firmly*) I am not in between. I am clearly one way.

> *Chaplain:* OK, so, it sounds like you are pretty clear about that.

> *Nate:* Yes, I am. But my family thinks it's a sin.

> *Chaplain:* They don't think it is OK?

> *Nate:* It is cultural, you know. And it is a religious thing for them, too. Do you think it is a sin to *think* this way? Or do you think it is only a sin to *act* this way? I mean, is it a sin that I think about guys, or is it just a sin if I were to do something with a guy.

> *Chaplain:* I believe that God created you the way you are. And I believe that God loves you no matter what you think or do.

> *Nate:* But do you think that it is a sin to think this way, or just a sin to act that way?

> *Chaplain:* Well, there are different teachings. Just like with human sexuality, there are churches that accept homosexuals but do not affirm homosexual relationships, and those churches do not think it is right to engage in same-sex relationships. And then there are churches that are affirming of same-sex relationships, as long as those relationships are loving. Those churches do not think it is a sin to think or act on homosexual feelings. (*pause*) And you do not

have to lose your faith in God because you realized that you like guys better.

Nate: I think I am really gay. I mean I think about guys. I am attracted to guys. That's just how it is for me.

Chaplain: Yes, this is how God made you. And God loves you the way you are.

Nate: OK. (*Pause*) But, you know, my family doesn't approve. Maybe when I go to college I might find people to talk to and people to be with. I can't tell my family now.

Chaplain: Yes, right now might not be the best time to tell your family. In the future, when you have moved out, there might be a better time to find people who are like you. And, you know, it might be a process. It might take a few years to figure it all out. You don't have to do it all now.

Nate: Yes, that's what I'm thinking. When I go away to college, you know.

Chaplain: You know who you are. And when the time is right you can decide whom you want to tell.

Nate: Yes, I think that is a good plan. I don't have to do anything right now. I just tell them I am too busy to date.

Chaplain: Right now you feel like you can make a compromise. And one day you might negotiate this compromise differently.

Nate: Yes. (*He seems relaxed, less awkward and more centered.*)

Chaplain: Do you ever talk to God about any of this?

Nate: Not so much. But I say my prayers. And I am a Eucharistic minister.

Chaplain: The practices of the Roman Catholic Church are important to you?

Nate: Yes. And I pray.

Chaplain: (*pause*) Would you like for us to say a prayer together?

Nate: (*Appearing more withdrawn.*) Yes.

Chaplain: We don't have to.

Nate: No, I think it would be OK to say a prayer.

Chaplain: What are you praying for as you leave here today?

Nate: (*Solemnly, looking down.*) For me to keep taking the medication and to go see the therapist.

Chaplain: To take your medication and to see your therapist.

Nate: And to stay on track with what the team told me to do.

Chaplain: And to stay on track. Anything else?

Nate: No, that's about it.

Chaplain: Nate, may God hear you and surround you with God's grace. Amen.

Nate: (*Perplexed, smiling.*) Amen.

Chaplain: So, what do you think? Are you ready to go?

Nate: Yeah, I think I am ready.

Chaplain: May God bless you and keep you always.

Nate: Thank you, chaplain.

Discussion

This holistic and spiritual assessment uses Fitchett's (1993) 7×7 model for spiritual assessment. Fitchett's model is based on a 'functional' approach, which emphasizes 'how a person makes meaning in his or her life' over the specific, 'substantive' content of the meaning (Fitchett 1993, p.40). The model considers seven holistic dimensions: medical; psychological; psychosocial; family systems; ethnic and cultural; societal issues; and spiritual. The final dimension is explored further in terms of: beliefs and meaning; vocation and consequences; experience and emotion; courage and growth; ritual and practice; community; and authority and guidance (Fitchett 1993). The aim is a holistic and spiritual assessment. But I also draw on Pargament's work on positive and negative religious/spiritual coping (Pargament 1997; Pargament, Feuille and Burdzy 2011), defining coping 'as efforts to understand and deal with life stressors in ways related to the sacred' (Pargament *et al.* 2011, p.52). This approach accounts for both the helpful and harmful effects of religious coping. Religious coping includes 'the search for meaning, intimacy with others, identity, control, anxiety-reduction, transformation, as well as the search for the sacred or spirituality itself' (Pargament *et al.* 2011, pp.52–53). It involves 'behaviors, emotions, relationships, and cognitions' (Pargament *et al.* 2011, p.53) that are based on a person's basic orienting system, which is the interpretive lens through which a person comes to understand the world. Faced with major life stressors, a person's orienting system is either conserved or transformed (Pargament 1997). 'No rule determines whether conserving or transforming our views is more helpful: either one can be helpful or harmful, depending on the person and the stressors faced' (Hartz 2005).

Holistic assessment

In addition to the patient's medical information, an appreciation of Nate's situation needs to take into account psychological, psychosocial, familial, ethnocultural and social factors (Fitchett 1993).

PSYCHOLOGICAL FACTORS

Nate stated that his 'fake life' was meaningless. Theories about 'coming out' describe a process of psychological integration. Newman and Muzzonigro (1993) describe three stages: sensitization; awareness with confusion, denial, guilt and shame; and acceptance. In the hospital, Nate was offered non-judgmental acceptance, empathic understanding and hope for a time in life when his current struggles could be overcome.

As Nate was searching for options for a spiritually and psychologically more authentic and healthier life, he became quite anxious. Nate's psychiatrist recalled a poignant moment for which I was not present. Encouraged to think about a future in which he could live his identity authentically by joining like-minded persons, Nate stated, 'Look, I am sitting in this chair. This chair is my family, my religion, my culture and my community. You are asking me to join these people over there that are more like me. But you do not understand. If I do this, I have to leave my chair.' Nate's anxiety centered on him and his family being ostracized by the Dominican community, both in the United States and in the Dominican Republic. The team's respectful, open and accepting attitude helped ease Nate's anxiety and sadness.

PSYCHOSOCIAL FACTORS

Nate was a high school student at a conservative Roman Catholic School. He worked as a cashier at a supermarket after school until late at night. Although his grades were initially good, they had recently deteriorated. His mother's cousin described him as a 'good' kid; however, since he had turned 18 years old, her attempts to discipline him were futile. Recently, he had not slept more than 5 hours a night due to consuming energy drinks throughout the day. With a distant history of being bullied in school, he was socially isolated and without friends. He stated that he felt unattractive and awkward most of the time. He did not smoke, drink alcohol or use drugs. He also denied hallucinations or feeling that he was possessed. The cousin of Nate's mother was convinced that the reason for Nate's difficulties were his struggles adjusting to life in the United States, particularly without his mother, who had raised him and with whom he was very close.

FAMILIAL FACTORS

Having worked on a psychiatric unit in the Dominican Republic, when Nate's mother learned of her son's inpatient psychiatric stay, she was horrified and advised against it. Traditionally, Dominicans may feel that therapeutic help is a waste of time, or that it is needed only by people who are seriously disturbed (McGoldrick, Giordano and Garcia-Preto 2005). Dominican parents can be protective and fearful, limiting their children's freedom. Possibly Nate's family was also fearful of his acculturation, which may have been faster than that of his extended family. While Nate's isolation was a source of concern, it is not uncommon for Dominican adolescents to be isolated from same-sex peers. Sexual education and open conversation about matters of sexuality are rare in Dominican families (McGoldrick *et al.* 2005). Due to a strong orientation towards traditional and conservative values, there are clear expectations and pressures around gender role, family values and religious beliefs (McGoldrick *et al.* 2005). Further intensifying the conflict, Nate had experienced his father's verbal and physical abuse of his mother as a child. While distant from his father, Nate was adamant about protecting his father from the shame associated with his son's sexual identity. Given this context, Nate's engagement in inpatient psychiatric treatment was quite remarkable. His agreement to conditional voluntary status demonstrated some differentiation from his family as well as insight into his need for psychiatric care and emotional support.

ETHNOCULTURAL FACTORS

Dominicans are the fourth largest group of Latinos in the United States. They maintain ties to their country of origin and tend to develop a sense of dual identity (McGoldrick *et al.* 2005). Nate's father and mother, though separated, resided in the Dominican Republic. He and his sister were chosen to immigrate and avail themselves of opportunities in the United States. His mother's cousin fulfilled a parenting role, aided by a close-knit Dominican community. Church attendance and social gatherings were aimed at maintaining the Dominican cultural, social and religious identity. His mother's cousin, with whom Nate lived, engaged in daily prayer and devotions at home in which Nate participated. He enjoyed singing in the church choir and was a senior in a conservative Roman

Catholic high school. His involvement in the Roman Catholic practices of his family, school and community provided structure and continuity to his social, cultural and family identity. The hierarchical organization of the church corresponded to the expectation of obedience to elders in the family. However, given that the average income of Dominicans is the lowest per capita in the United States (McGoldrick *et al.* 2005), it is understandable that thinking positively about his future and confidence in a better life were hard to come by for Nate.

SOCIAL FACTORS

Nate's story unfolded in the context of social forces. The professional psychiatric community today considers same-sex attractions and behaviors as non-pathological variants of human sexuality. The Roman Catholic Church, while accepting of homosexuality, views homosexual acts as sinful and necessitating healing (see USCCB 1994, paragraphs 2357–2359). Attitudes of American Catholics have been changing, with 49% affirming this teaching in 2003 versus 33% in 2013, and 43% seeing no conflict between their religious beliefs and homosexuality (Pew Research Center 2013). Additionally, while 64% of Americans look to God for strength, support and guidance when faced with major life stressors, among American psychiatrists only 36% were found to engage in religious coping (Curlin *et al.* 2005, pp.631–632). These findings add a layer of complexity to the psychiatric treatment of patients whose struggles have a significant religious component.

Spiritual assessment

The spiritual assessment focuses on the following dimensions: belief and meaning; vocation and obligation; experience and emotion; courage and growth; ritual and practice; community; as well as authority and guidance (Fitchett 1993).

BELIEF AND MEANING

Nate had a good understanding of Roman Catholic teachings. The religious and cultural prohibition against living his homosexual identity caused him profound, potentially chronic religious struggle. When his family requested a Bible and the Sacrament of Confession, Nate's choice was either to comply, and conserve his family's orienting system, or to begin the work of adjusting his belief system, as many Latino, Roman Catholic, homosexual adolescents tend to do (García, Gray-Stanley and Ramirez-Valles 2008). Developing his own belief system carried the risk of losing family and communal contexts that met Nate's needs for food, shelter, security, family connection, community and education. While looking for meaning and direction, he was also seeking comfort and the assurance of God's love.

VOCATION AND OBLIGATION

Nate felt obligated to contribute financially to his family. What Griffith (2012) terms reciprocal altruism offered him a sense of belonging to a community and ensured that he was taken care of. In turn, Nate contributed to his family financially, and to his community religiously by serving as Eucharistic minister. His duties left little space for his visions of his future, and his emerging ability to imagine a meaningful personal and vocational life caused him fear and conflict. Increasingly, thinking positively about his future also offered Nate the potential for transforming his current blueprint for his life.

EXPERIENCE AND EMOTION

Nate suffered from significant self-hate, shame, guilt, isolation, inauthenticity, sadness, fear and hopelessness. With the courage of despair, Nate had attempted suicide to resolve the conflict in which he found himself. His survival opened a tenuous possibility for him to attend to his personal, emotional and spiritual growth. His inpatient stay offered help in learning new coping strategies. While he seemed to enter into some questioning, there was little evidence that he was actually transforming his religious/spiritual framework. His personal spirituality was overall hidden, as if to help him make the necessary compromises that might carry him beyond the current crisis; however, his willingness to engage cognitively in different strategies to resolve his conflict was important progress.

COURAGE AND GROWTH

Traditionally, Dominicans grow up with little room for rebellion during puberty and adolescence. Reasoning, explanations and negotiations are not valued as a tool in childrearing. *Simpatia*, a key value for Dominicans (McGoldrick *et al.* 2005), calls for good manners, common courtesy and the expectation of conformity. Additionally, Nate was unable to experience a self apart from what others were telling him or asking of him. His meaning-making system was what Kegan (1982) refers to as the *interpersonal* stage of the mind. Characteristic for this stage, the locus of authority was in others – family, religious community, medical team. Nate did not yet have an inner author to define his identity. He was not mature enough to express himself and, as expected at this stage of development, it was difficult for him to tolerate competing perspectives. For this reason, my interventions emphasized empathy in order to build an alliance and a shared sense of self. Support for different ways of meaning-making seemed developmentally appropriate; however, expectations that Nate would resolve the conflict between different belief and value systems were unrealistic. Not resolving the conflict also protected him at this vulnerable moment in his life from facing profound loss.

RITUAL AND PRACTICE

It was the family, not Nate himself, who requested a Bible and a Roman Catholic priest visit. In my mind, Nate's vulnerability to having his religious/spiritual beliefs disrespected was similar to a patient who is not able to speak for themselves, with family members attempting to 'save' or convert the patient by requesting religious/spiritual rituals in life-threatening clinical situations. Additionally, in my experience, patients who have survived a suicide attempt frequently ask for the Roman Catholic priest to confess their 'sin'. Nate did not speak of a reason for confession, other than his religious struggle regarding his sexuality.

COMMUNITY

Nate was a part of several communities: family, school, church and ethnic community; however, his participation in these communities had come to feel inauthentic to him, resulting in isolation and fear.

AUTHORITY AND GUIDANCE

Reportedly, the cousin of Nate's mother thought that Nate was possessed. She felt that Nate urgently needed the healing offered through Scripture and sacraments. His family saw the Roman Catholic priest as an important authority who could bring healing. Relinquishing his own authority, Nate was willing to go along, which also had the potential of conserving and deepening his religious struggle. In our interactions, I was aware of the potential power dynamics. It was likely that Nate saw me as aligned with the medical team. I was aware of possible compliance on his part, while aiming at honoring *his* religious/spiritual autonomy and supporting *his* religious/spiritual needs. In our relational space, Nate negotiated giving me authority and taking authority himself as well. He was increasingly present and alive in our conversations.

Interventions and outcomes

My interventions in the first encounter responded to Nate's presenting need to comply with his family's request for a Bible. *Respeto*, another key Dominican concept and attitude (McGoldrick *et al.* 2005), helped me to establish a relationship with this young man, and I offered psychoeducational interventions respectfully. I communicated respect for Nate's religious/spiritual identity and normalized that certain religious/spiritual attitudes were helpful for some people but not helpful for others. I respected Nate's need for rest in a time of vulnerability and crisis, and this contributed to his sense of safety on the unit.

In the second encounter, I communicated interest in Nate beyond any religious/spiritual issues. Through non-threatening, non-judgmental, empathic inquiry, trust was established. Normalizing and generalizing of Nate's developmental tasks reduced his sense of isolation. I engaged his hopelessness by affirming his abilities, encouraging his plans and empowering him to envision his future the way he would want it to be. Nate was invited to imagine himself looking back on this time in his life, when the conflict was successfully resolved.

In the last and most significant encounter, Nate was invited to engage his underlying religious struggle. Exploration of the request for confession allowed for discussion of Nate's identity and beliefs, his understanding of the Roman Catholic teachings and a potential renegotiation of his relationship to those teachings. Additional education about human sexuality and the teachings of different religious denominations opened a wider horizon for his struggle. Support for Nate's religious autonomy and development of his 'inner author' made it possible to imagine different orienting systems, which in the future might allow for positive coping in the presence of continuing stressors. Shame and self-deprecation were countered with the assurance of God's love for God's creation (i.e. Nate himself). The outcome was a visibly calmer demeanor in the patient. I supported Nate to express his needs in relationship with a power transcending the constraints of religious dogma, by inviting him to formulate his prayer requests. Rather than adding to or reformulating his petitions, I empowered Nate and offered an experience of simply talking to God in human ways. The prayer also reaffirmed the need for psychiatric follow-up and treatment compliance. Mindful of the important transition on the day of discharge, a blessing offered reassurance at a time that usually generates anxiety.

These interventions offered ways of developing an orienting belief system that was different from Nate's cultural, familial and religious context. Interventions were aimed at greater flexibility of cognition, beliefs and moral values, opening the possibility of imagining a future beyond the current crisis and conflict. In the course of the third encounter, Nate came out to himself and claimed his sexual identity with a religious person. This was significant, even though arguably only the beginning of a much longer journey of self-acceptance and renegotiation of meaning-making.

Conclusion

Nate's personality test revealed cognitive inflexibility, suspiciousness and difficulty with flexible problem solving. My interventions attempted to build trust, particularly with a person representing religion/ spirituality. At the same time, Nate's ability to make use of these new ways of engaging with his religious struggle and conflicted orienting system were limited. Nate did not express to me feelings of guilt related to his suicide attempt, even though the protective effects of religion for suicidal patients are well documented. Additionally, Nate was about to rejoin his familiar environment, including the orienting system of his family, culture and religion of origin. Involving a Roman Catholic priest may have been beneficial. In conversations with Roman Catholic priest colleagues, my interventions with Nate were affirmed, suggesting that a priest might have engaged Nate in similar ways. It is impossible to judge whether absolution from a Roman Catholic priest would have been more healing, less or the same to Nate. There was also a risk that a chaplaincy intervention through a Roman Catholic priest may have further exacerbated Nate's struggles.

Given the relatively short hospitalization, there may have been opportunities missed by not intentionally bridging Nate's inpatient psychiatric stay with his family and religious community. Beyond managing the acute crisis, this work needed to continue in outpatient treatment. Goals for Nate's outpatient treatment included exploration of sexual identity, self-esteem and considerations for his future. Continued psychopharmacological assistance was aimed to help move toward flexible coping and reduction of catastrophic, self-deprecatory thoughts.

When religious/spiritual issues are part of the stressors leading to or contributing to a patient's psychiatric illness, chaplaincy involvement is a crucial part of the overall treatment approach. Earlier and more fully integrated care across different patient care areas may be beneficial to patients. Clinicians seem generally reluctant to call upon the chaplain; however, when religion presents serious and life-threatening risks, the chaplain is the expert to help negotiate religious struggle. Chaplains offer cultural and religious expertise, which may be key in negotiating the patient's culture with the team's culture.

References

Angst, J., Angst, F. and Strassen, H.H. (1999) 'Suicide risk in patients with major depressive disorder.' *Journal of Clinical Psychiatry 60*, 2, 57–62.

Aronow, E., Altman Weiss, K. and Reznikoff, M. (2001) *A Practical Guide to the Thematic Apperception Test: The TAT in Clinical Practice*. Philadelphia, PA: Taylor and Francis.

Curlin, F.A., Lanton, J.D., Roach, C.J., Sellergren, S.A. and Marshall, H.C. (2005) 'Religious characteristics of U.S. physicians: A national survey.' *Journal of General Internal Medicine 20*, 7, 629–634.

Fitchett, G. (1993) *Assessing Spiritual Needs: A Guide for Caregivers*. Minneapolis, MN: Augsbrug Fortress.

García, D.I., Gray-Stanley, J. and Ramirez-Valles, J. (2008) '"The priest obviously doesn't know that I'm gay": The religious and spiritual journeys of Latino gay men.' *Journal of Homosexuality 55*, 3, 411–436.

Griffith, L.L. (2012) 'Psychiatry and mental health treatment.' In M. Cobb, C.M. Puchalski and B. Rumbold (eds) *Oxford Textbook of Spirituality in Healthcare*. Oxford: Oxford University Press, 227–233.

Hartz, G. (2005) *Spirituality and Mental Health: Clinical Applications*. Binghampton, NY: The Haworth Pastoral Press.

Kegan, R. (1982) *The Evolving Self: Problem and Process in Human Development*. Cambridge, MA: Harvard University Press.

Khan, A., Leventhan, R.M., Khan, S. and Brown, W.A. (2002) 'Suicide risk in patients with anxiety disorders: A meta-analysis of the FDA database.' *Journal of Affective Disorders 68*, 2–3, 183–190.

McGoldrick, M., Giordano, J. and Garcia-Preto, N. (eds) (2005) *Ethnicity and Family Therapy* (3rd edn). New York, NY: The Guilford Press.

Morey, L.C. (2007) *Personality Assessment Inventory (PAI)*. Lutz, FL: Psychological Assessment Resources.

Newman, B.S. and Muzzonigro, P.N. (1993) 'The effects of traditional family values on the coming out process of gay male adolescents.' *Adolescence 28*, 109, 213–226.

Pargament, K. (1997) *The Psychology of Religion and Coping: Theory, Research, and Practice*. New York, NY: The Guilford Press.

Pargament, K., Feuille, M. and Burdzy, D. (2011) 'The Brief RCOPE: Current psychometric status of a short measure of religious coping.' *Religions 2*, 1, 51–76.

Pew Research Center (2013) 'Section 3: Religious Beliefs and Views of Homosexuality.' Available at www.people-press.org/2013/06/06/section-3-religious-belief-and-views-of-homosexuality, accessed on 4 July 2014.

Razani, J., Murcia, G., Tabares, J. and Wong, J. (2006) 'The effects of culture on WASI Test performance in ethnically diverse individuals.' *The Clinical Neuropsychologist 21*, 5, 776–788.

USCCB (1994) *Catechism of the Catholic Church*. Washington, DC: United States Catholic Conference Inc; Libreria Editrice Vaticana.

Wechsler, D. (1955) *Manual for the Wechsler Adult Intelligence Scale*. Oxford: Psychological Corp.

Chapter 9
Critical Response to Psychiatric Case Studies

A Chaplain/Psychologist's Perspective

Graeme D. Gibbons

I am an ordained minister of the Uniting Church in Australia and an accredited clinical pastoral education (CPE) supervisor. I was a chaplain and Director of the Austin Hospital Clinical Pastoral Education Center in Melbourne for 32 years. Following my retirement in 2007, I established a small private practice as a psychologist and psychotherapist. I am currently President of the Empathink Association of Psychoanalytic Self-Psychology, a member organization of the International Association of Self-Psychology. In thinking about how to respond to these cases, I have limited myself to one major theme within each.

Yesuto: Transgeneration of trauma

I think Chaplain Ratcliffe has done a wonderful job of exploring the ethnocultural dimensions involved in Yesuto's case. At home, Yesuto was going out of his mind, and on presentation in hospital he communicates his fear of being hounded by witches. When Chaplain Ratcliffe took an empathic interest in Yesuto's 'deserved suffering' and asked 'Why has this witch chosen to "target" you?' he responded, 'I am so frightened. I am frightened for my baby. I think that he is going to die when he is 8 years old.' At this point in the remembered written document there is a change in Yesuto's affect and tone.

Yesuto went on to tell Chaplain Ratcliffe what I thought was an important detail: that his parents were visiting from Nigeria. Not only did they reinforce the witchcraft theory, they were witch-like by reminding Yesuto of their preferred model of childcare. I wonder whether Yesuto's intensity and internal conflict comes from his fear of displeasing or offending his parents' expectations. A significant addition to the intensity of his conflict was revealed when he told Chaplain Ratcliffe his wife had recently given birth to their first child, and his parents were warning him not to love his son 'too much'. This followed the belief his parents and grandparents held that loving a child too much would increase the likelihood of the child suffering harm in some way.

Momentarily, Chaplain Ratcliffe's focus and understanding of Yesuto's subjective experience waned as she put forward a theory of why they might think that way. I appreciated the way in which Chaplain Ratcliffe recovered and returned her focus to Yesuto. She engaged Yesuto around his own childhood with an enlightened and open question: 'What happened to you when you were 8 years old?' Yesuto's answer drew a picture of a traumatized child and a wider picture of transgenerational trauma. Yesuto's parents' preferred model of childcare, which set a limit on the love they expressed in their attachment to their children, was not benign but in fact, to a greater or lesser degree, a traumatizing model.

I was left with some questions about the trauma Yesuto experienced during his going back and forth from home to boarding school. How does an 8-year-old child, knowing his parents don't love him too much, cope with strange authority figures at boarding school? Was the school environment healthy or was there abuse, either physical, emotional or sexual? We do know that he was now faced with the insistence from his parents that he follow their pattern of childcare in his care of his newborn child. I remembered one of my CPE supervisors and mentors who worked for a long time in a large psychiatric hospital sharing that from his clinical experience, patients who had foreboding premonitions about their children's destiny had often been traumatized themselves as a child.

Clearly, from what he had said to Chaplain Ratcliffe, Yesuto had been traumatized as a child at the age of 8 years, and in an ongoing way. It is relational trauma that initiates the co-creation of complex systems of pathological accommodation. (I say more about this in response to the case of Nate.)

In her reflective appraisal, Chaplain Ratcliffe claimed, 'as is the case with cognitive behavioural therapy, I focused on the "here and now".' However, the case opened up when she went beyond her cognitive behavioural therapy approach and took Yesuto back to his past with her empathic question, 'What happened to you when you were 8 years old?'

From my perspective as a psychoanalytical self-psychologist, Yesuto was dealing with feelings, emotions and attitudes embedded in areas of the brain, such as the basal ganglia and the amygdala, that are responsible for implicit procedural memory, and are not easily changed by logic and cognitive thinking, but can be regulated over time by regular empathic understanding and responsiveness.

From my perspective as a chaplain, the patient's subjective experience is very important. Sometimes chaplains understand concepts too concretely when it is better to understand them as metaphors. I thought that to be the case with Yesuto's witches. There are witches in Australia, the USA, England and Nigeria. They appear in families and communities in the form of demanding expectations. As a chaplain, minister and psychologist I have met them in the psyche of my patients, especially those who have been traumatized as children. Yesuto's parents and grandparents had been witch-like in their model of childcare. I suggest it would have been helpful if Yesuto had been followed up with either longer-term psychotherapy from an empathic therapist or through the support of a Christian community, who could remind Yesuto each day that 'I never heard the voice of Jesus say, don't love your child too much', not only for his sake but also for the sake of his newly born child.

June: A theological attitude to suicide

June's case engaged me as a theologian. It clearly introduces the theme of suicide and attitudes held to suicide. In considering the case, it does seem clear that June had requested a chaplain to speak about the issue of her attempting to take her own life and the badness she experienced about her attempt that went wrong. I think the chaplain had been called in as a theologian. It does seem from Chaplain Swift's introduction that the referral was a good fit, as he was an ordained Anglican priest completing a Masters in Theology and had some formal training in counselling skills. When they met, June asked, 'Can we talk somewhere privately?'

June, like many of her contemporaries, had once been connected to a church but had dropped out, yet she still held belief in some of the Church's teachings from her childhood that had been based in superstition and fear. Psychologist of religion, Kenneth Pargament, has described how in the face of life crises such poorly integrated religious beliefs can contribute to religious/spiritual struggles that put patients at risk of poor health outcomes (Pargament 2007). Some old beliefs that are overwhelming and negative are held onto and do not provide a health-giving spirituality.

As I read Chaplain Swift's account of his work with June I recollected some theological views about suicide as a pastoral issue. My views were shaped by reading theologians Paul Tillich and Dietrich Bonhoeffer, and by James Hillman, analyst and former Director of Studies at the C.G. Jung institute in Zurich, when I was a theological student 40 years ago.

Hillman's enchanting book, *Suicide and the Soul* (Hillman 1964), in which he challenges and dismisses the approaches taken to suicide by sociology, law, theology and mental health, intrigued me. In all these approaches he thought suicide was prejudged and understood only as a symptom or sign of alienation to be approached with a strong determination 'to save life' (Hillman 1964, p.20). June was so angry with the medical profession for having brought her back from death. She had planned her death well, even taking the caution of sending second class mail to ensure that the police, rather than a few friends or neighbours, would discover her body.

June's emphysema was slowly killing her. She felt alone and abandoned, and just wanted to be with the person she loved. Hillman (1964) advocated giving recognition to the states of the soul, which the person concerned is undergoing, so that they may be lived consciously by the patient. June seemed to recognize and understand what was going on for her and, when the staff could not confirm what was going on in her love for her partner, Chaplain Swift provided the kind of confirmatory relationship to June that Hillman advocated.

In Tillich's view, an attempt to take your own life is a dimension of despair. 'Despair', he said, 'is an ultimate or "boundary-line" situation. One cannot go beyond it. Its nature is indicated in the etymology of the word despair – without hope. No way out into the future appears' (Tillich 1952, p.61).

Tillich believed that the situation of despair can be met in three ways: first, it can be met with courage, which is the self-affirmation to live 'in spite of despair' (p.70); second, it can be met with an escape into neurosis; third, it can be met with an attempt to get rid of one's self. June had been encountering the boundary line of despair and had attempted to get rid of herself.

It was Bonhoeffer (1955) who provided a theological gem when in his reformed theology he pointed out that suicide, while certainly taking place in a state of despair, actually originates from our freedom, which makes a person attempt to put things right themselves. For Bonhoeffer, the only wrong people like June commit is that of lack of faith, and this because she sought to justify herself (something that is part of the human condition) rather than trust in the living God.

June initiated the theological question: 'Listen, I need to ask you something. Because I've tried to kill myself, do you think God will keep me apart from the person I love, you know, in the life-after?' Chaplain Swift seemed to struggle to reply.

June's statement was clear: 'I need to know what you really believe.' It does sound like she wanted to know where the chaplain stood about the issue of suicide. Chaplain Swift took a standpoint; he shared his view that 'God isn't vindictive' and doesn't punish people for doing what she has done.

If I place myself in June's situation, while I welcomed Chaplain Swift's response I would have liked him to be a little stronger about how he felt and where he stood. If I was in June's place, I would be asking, 'Do you have a word for me, in my situation of despair and taking the responsibility on myself, and loving another woman more than some think is reasonable?' I would like someone to be able to integrate Tillich, Bonhoeffer and Hillman into a succinct statement. I would like a chaplain to say something like:

> June, I think this is one area of belief that parts of the church has in the past got seriously wrong. I believe you have experienced the loss of someone whose value has been extremely important to you. You were in deep despair, and one of the ways people try to escape from despair is to try foolishly to make it right themselves, to take it on themselves. That act is often a cry for help. I would like to work with you to try to understand how important it is for you to join your friend, even if that means later you try to complete what you didn't succeed with this time. I would like you and I to be clear about your love of this woman, a love that is so powerful.

Nate: Systems of pathological accommodation

Using the 7×7 model for spiritual assessment (Fitchett 1993), Chaplain Zollfrank wrote an excellent psychological section of her holistic assessment of Nate. She succinctly reports Nate felt that his 'fake life' was meaningless but that he was stuck where he was. Chaplain Zollfrank reports Nate's response to a frank discussion with his psychiatrist about his homosexuality and his fear of coming out with his family, in which he stated, 'Look, I am sitting in this chair. This chair is my family, my religion, my culture and my community. You are asking me to join these people over there that are more like me. But you do not understand. If I do this, I have to leave my chair.'

This statement engaged me as a self-psychologist who has been absorbing the influence of the late Bernie Brandchaft, over the many years he explored his understanding of the concept of 'systems of pathological accommodation' (Beandchaft, Doctors and Sorter 2010, p.193). Pathological accommodation involves co-participants, one partner who expects the other to adjust who they are to their expectations. It begins when the child accommodates to the expectations of parents and other caregivers. It continues when adults accommodate to the expectations of various authorities that come along. As Nate put it about his relationship with his family, 'I mean, I'll just go with it. They seem to be adamant, and I don't really care.'

It is a process in which there are partners. I appreciated the care and patience Chaplain Zollfrank invested in helping Nate to make his own decision about calling or not calling a priest, and either going to confession or having a conversation with her. Professional caregivers can also fall into the role of the partner in the relationship who holds the expectations that must be met. Chaplain Zollfrank avoided a partnership that was unhealthy or pathological. She did not have unrelenting and unremitting expectations which Nate had to accommodate or honour at considerable cost to his self-agency.

The first sign of others' expectations that Nate should toe the line was the family's request that he be given a Bible; the second came on the day he left the hospital with the directive that he see a priest. Chaplain Zollfrank named the issue for Nate when she said, 'I think your problem is that you do not know what to say to your family, if you do not see a priest.' Nate experienced Chaplain Zollfrank's empathic understanding and reflected this in his response, delivered with a spark in his eye, 'Well, yes, that's just it.' 'The needs and feelings of the parent are then privileged by the child at the expense of the child's authentic self experience' (Brandchaft, Doctors and Sorter 2010, p.3).

I liked the way in which Chaplain Zollfrank opened up the issue of human sexuality by sharing how she thought about it being on a continuum from heterosexual to those who are homosexual and are attracted to persons of their own sex. Nate is very clear in indicating that he is at the 'gay' end of the continuum, and he is also clear that he is not ready to tell his family.

I really agree with Chaplain Zollfrank's stance with Nate when she writes, 'In attempts to support him, it was important to remain attentive to Nate's conflict, rather than trying to resolve it prematurely.'

Chaplain Zollfrank notes that physical signs of fear and conflict intensified when Nate nervously talked about his family, which was 'so different' from him, wanted him to 'be like them' and 'did not understand him'. He was 'ruminative, vague and fidgety'.

Structures of pathological accommodation are enduring life patterns. They endure through childhood, adolescence, adulthood and into old age. They are passed on across generations from parents to children. Chaplains, pastoral practitioners and others who work in mental health need to be alert to such patterns developing in their treatment relationships with their patients.

Conclusion

In each of these cases, I thought the actual work was well done by the chaplains. They were professional, caring and reflective before, during and following the practice. The specific nature of these cases reminds us of the importance of being specific in our chaplaincy case reports, and that responsiveness within a chaplain-patient dyad is inescapably reciprocal, that is, both chaplain and patient give and receive. At the conclusion of this response, I want to affirm this body of work. I am sure it will provide helpful education to a new generation of chaplains and pastoral practitioners.

References

Brandchaft, B., Doctors, S. and Sorter, D. (2010) *Toward an Emancipatory Psychoanalysis: Brandchaft's Intersubjective Vision*. New York, NY: Routledge.

Bonhoeffer, D. (1955) *Ethics*. London: SCM Press.

Fitchett, G. (1993) *Assessing Spiritual Needs: A Guide for Caregivers*. Minneapolis, MN: Augsburg Fortress.

Hillman, J. (1964) *Suicide and the Soul*. London: Hodder and Stoughton.

Pargament, K.I. (2007) *Spiritually Integrated Psychotherapy: Understanding and Addressing the Sacred*. New York, NY: The Guilford Press.

Tillich, P. (1952) *The Courage To Be*. London: Fontana.

Chapter 10

Critical Response to Psychiatric Case Studies

A Psychiatrist's Perspective

Warren Kinghorn

Modern Western medical systems, organized according to hierarchies of experts who administer various 'specialty' practices, often consider healthcare chaplains to be a type of specialist. In the paradigm of medical specialization, chaplains are understood as specialists of a particular domain, sometimes termed 'spiritual care'. Physicians and other clinicians, not generally trained in spiritual matters, are often glad to hand over spiritual care to experts who do have such training, particularly when the experts involved are health system employees and therefore accountable to the values and standards of the healthcare system. Chaplains, in turn, play an exceedingly important role in attending to the humanistic gap created when bioscientific medical practices come into contact with the complex, context-constituted lives of people who are sick.

When spiritual questions and concerns arise in *response* to particular forms of illness – as, for example, when a person with newly diagnosed metastatic cancer questions why God would allow such a thing to happen – the specialization model of spiritual care works quite straightforwardly. Medical experts can treat the person's disease, while chaplains can attend to the spiritual questions that arise in response to the disease. Actual cases, of course, are often complex, but the basic model is familiar: physicians treat disease, and chaplains attend to patients and families as they cope with and respond to the experience of illness.

There are many problems with this way of understanding the role differentiation of physicians and chaplains, but the model becomes untenable in the context of the care of people with mental health problems. Religious and spiritual concerns, after all, are frequently woven into the fabric of mental health problems, making mental health problems the kind of things that they are. To be sure, spiritual concerns can arise in response to the experience of mental disorder, as when a person newly diagnosed with Alzheimer'-type dementia fears what the future will bring. But spiritual concerns can sometimes stand as a *cause* of mental health problems, as when a soldier's religiously motivated guilt over acts done in war lead to a syndrome nearly indistinguishable from post-traumatic stress disorder; or mental health problems may simply *be* spiritual concerns, as in the case of a person with 'religious delusions'. This interweaving of spiritual matters into the fabric of mental health problems should call into question whether any sharp distinction between the 'psychiatric' and the 'spiritual' is either necessary or tenable.

This complex interweaving of spiritual matters into the fabric of mental health problems places chaplains in a correlatively complex relationship with other members of the multidisciplinary care team. Sometimes, for example, chaplains may be equipped not only to attend to a patient's response to mental health problems, but also to understand the mental health problems themselves more perceptively than the patient's medical providers. It would be nearly unthinkable, for example, for a chaplain on an inpatient oncology unit to challenge an oncologist about the accuracy of a particular cancer diagnosis. But it is not unthinkable – or, at least, *should* not be unthinkable – that a well-equipped chaplain might challenge a psychiatrist's core formulation of a particular patient's mental health problem. Chaplains might argue, for example, that what a psychiatrist labels 'depression' in a particular patient is best understood as unresolved shame, or that what a psychiatrist labels 'paranoia' in a particular patient is a contextually appropriate response to racism and neighborhood violence. Chaplains ought to be able to make these sort of arguments when necessary and appropriate.

This blurring of boundaries between medical care and spiritual care, however, poses challenges for the chaplain's relationship to psychiatrists and other team members. Some psychiatrists may welcome, and indeed even celebrate, deep collaboration with chaplains in a patient's care, but others will not, either as a result of ignorance about the sort of wisdom chaplains can bring or by actively resisting intrusion of the 'spiritual' into medical models of diagnosis and treatment. Chaplains further must contend with the sticky reality that for many patients, 'spirituality' is community- and tradition-mediated. Spiritual care therefore frequently requires chaplains to engage the communities and traditions that have formed patients to be the sorts of spiritual seekers that they are. Chaplains are usually ordained within particular religious communities and are sometimes expected to minister the presence of that community (i.e. the Catholic sacraments for a Catholic chaplain) to patients of the same faith background. But even when this is not the case, chaplains must often engage patients' particular faith traditions and communities while caring for them. When the commitments of a patient's formative faith tradition come into conflict with the commitments of the medical team, with the patient caught in the middle, the chaplain may feel pressure to take sides or to distance himself or herself both from the medical team and from the patient's faith community. Negotiating these pressures can be quite challenging, particularly in the spiritual care of people hospitalized for mental health problems. Chaplains are aligned through institutional affiliation and professional identity with the multidisciplinary care team, but they bear wisdom and insight that may challenge the core assumptions of more powerful clinicians on the team. Chaplains may or may not be aligned with the religious traditions and communities of which patients are a part, but they are nonetheless sometimes expected to stand in for those traditions while the patient is hospitalized. Furthermore, chaplains are, above all, aligned with the patient, who may well be caught between the demands of the medical care team and his or her formative religious community. How are chaplains to navigate such complex structural challenges?

Each of the insightful case studies provided by Chaplains Ratcliffe, Swift and Zollfrank features a patient with mental health problems who is torn among his or her formative religious tradition, the normative expectations of the medical care team and his or her own evolving sense of personal identity. Together, these case studies offer three complementary but distinct models for how chaplains might negotiate this complex three-way tension.

In her encounter with Yesuto, Chaplain Ratcliffe finds herself in a liminal space. She is a member of the multidisciplinary team and values her role as a specialist in 'the relation between faith, illness and the emotional conflicts that can arise in a person's thinking', and yet resists the medical language of psychosis that is used by the team to describe Yesuto's religious experience. Conversely, she shares Yesuto's Christian faith and his experience of immigration, but resists his belief in the power of witches and his emphasis on his own inadequacy and sinfulness. Although as a psychiatrist I am not able to conclude from the case description whether a diagnosis of psychosis or delusion was appropriate for Yesuto – that would require more information about Yesuto's thoughts, behavior and experience over time, including in the weeks and months prior to his hospitalization – I applaud the way that Chaplain Ratcliffe was able to leverage this creative tension in a way that, in the end, brought Yesuto closer to his own religious tradition and also enabled him to engage more effectively in his own medical care. The insistence of the medical team on pathologizing Yesuto's religious experience, without engaging it on Yesuto's own terms, may paradoxically have exacerbated not only his deep-seated feelings of shame and inadequacy but also his feelings of being persecuted, as he experienced himself as an alien in a hostile, power-wielding environment. (It is worth remembering, in this context, that the Gerasene man in the synoptic gospels named his oppressors *legion*, the transliterated Latin name of the imperial military units occupying Palestine at the time; see Mark 5:9.) In contrast, Chaplain Ratcliffe's invitation to Yesuto to speak openly and non-defensively about his religious beliefs, and to explore them without shame, provided much-needed space for him to consider them non-defensively and, eventually, to question them.

I applaud Chaplain Ratcliffe's general approach as well as her affirmation that 'people's spiritual or religious beliefs should not be interpreted as symptoms of disordered minds', though I would qualify that psychosis can indeed often take a specifically religious/spiritual form. But I fear that her well-placed commitment not to pathologize religious experience by recourse to medical models is somewhat undermined by the way that she pathologizes Yesuto's religious beliefs by recourse to psychological literature, as when she refers to a brand of religion and Christianity that 'was detrimental to mental well-being.' It is interesting to me that the conviction that Yesuto's religion was 'detrimental' led Chaplain Ratcliffe to be more directive and didactic than at other points of her encounter, pointing Yesuto to a series of biblical texts which focus on the unconditional love of God. Fortunately, Yesuto seemed to respond positively to this, without intensification of shame, but given his position as a patient and hers as a member of the multidisciplinary care team, what choice did he have but to agree with her?

In his encounter with June, Chaplain Swift also finds himself occupying an ambiguous and liminal space between the medical team and June's formative religious tradition, though in a different way. He is personally drawn to June, admiring her plain-spokenness and honesty, and seems intent neither to be a 'God-botherer', on one hand, nor an apostle of the multidisciplinary care team, on the other. Instead, he assumes the role of a confidante and priest, engaging June's spiritual concerns openly and frankly, celebrating Holy Communion with her, and becoming something of a confessor for her. This latter function, never named as such, is displayed in his decision not to disclose to the care team members that June was likely lying to them in the assessment meeting at which she was determined to be ready for discharge. He bears her burden in confidence, simultaneously strengthening her rapport with him and leaving him uneasy about her safety following discharge.

Chaplain Swift's decision not to disclose June's ongoing thoughts of suicide to the care team is deeply rooted in his pastoral relationship with her, but as he hints in his discussion of the case, it also represents a missed opportunity for interprofessional collaboration that could have proved beneficial to June, Chaplain Swift and the medical caregivers. Although breaking confidence with June would have threatened his pastoral relationship with her, Chaplain Swift could ideally have encouraged June to be honest about her feelings with the care team and, simultaneously, spoken to the care team members about his understanding of June's situation. Had June been honest with the team during the assessment meeting, this could have led to a straightforward discussion about June's hopes and fears that would have been helpful to all involved, with no need for secrets.

When June repeatedly speaks of suicide, Chaplain Swift wisely resolves not to go 'prospecting' by attempting to persuade her that she has reasons not to die. But his reluctance to dissuade her from suicide in any way, even suggesting that she might benefit from contemporary right-to-die laws being proposed in the UK, is puzzling. June's suffering stems not only from grief but from loneliness and isolation, and one response to such isolation, signified in the Holy Communion shared with her, is a caring community. It is good that a handoff of care was made to a local cleric when June was discharged, but might there have been more ways to encourage new forms of participation in local parish life?

The ambiguous and liminal space that chaplains occupy with respect to medical care teams and patients' formative religious communities is especially evident in Chaplain Zollfrank's intriguing case study, though she aligns herself more closely with the medical care team and more distantly from the patient's religious community than either Chaplain

Ratcliffe or Chaplain Swift. Chaplain Zollfrank agrees with the dominant judgment of the medical team that Nate is likely gay, that he is not yet able to speak openly about this and that his Catholic faith is an obstacle to his ability to name and claim his authentic sexual identity. Because of this, given Nate's claim that his request to see a priest for confession/absolution originated with his family and not with him, Chaplain Zollfrank steers Nate away from seeing a priest, engaging him instead in a conversation in which he is able to acknowledge, perhaps for only the second time, that he is 'really gay' and 'attracted to guys'. Her candid, matter-of-fact, non-defensive style empowered Nate to speak freely and to develop trust in their relationship. Nate clearly trusted her despite their differences of age, gender and culture – a testament to Chaplain Zollfrank's ability to establish an open, honest relationship with him.

Chaplain Zollfrank's decision to challenge Nate on his request for a Catholic priest, stemming from her concern that Nate's Catholic religious background was contributing to his hopelessness and suicidality, is understandable but nonetheless represents a missed opportunity for Nate to engage more deeply with his Catholic faith while on the inpatient unit (as Chaplain Zollfrank herself suggests in her discussion). While it is true that present-day Catholic teaching regards same-sex sexual acts (but not same-sex desires) as sinful, it is also true that Nate is a deeply formed Catholic. Catholicism is the 'chair' that will continue to affect him, mediated not only through the church but through his family and culture. Why not, then, allow Nate to meet with a priest and then remain available to process that engagement with him, with a possible subsequent conversation with the priest also? Although individual priests would differ in their ability to engage Nate's deepest concerns effectively, and would also differ in their own views of homosexuality, involving Catholic clergy would help Nate to experience his emerging understanding of sexual identity *internally* to his journey as a Catholic Christian, and not externally, through a narrative of identity and orientation encouraged by the medical care team and its protestant chaplain.

There is, to be sure, the possibility that Nate could be harmed were he to see a priest for confession. If, for example, a priest were immediately to refer Nate to a 'reparative therapy' program with the promise that his sexual-desire patterns would change, then the medical team would be right to express concern and alarm (APA 2009). In our time, however, such a referral is increasingly unlikely. But harm can also come when clinicians (and chaplains) overstate scientific consensus about sexual orientation and therefore widen possible rifts between patients and their religious/cultural communities. Chaplain Zollfrank's assurance to Nate that 'this is how God made you' strongly connotes that Nate's same-sex sexual orientation is innate. But the research literature is not so clear. There are no unambiguous answers within the scientific literature regarding the genesis of sexual orientation and identity, except that sexuality emerges, like all complex forms of human experience and behavior, within interconnected matrices of biology, environment and culture (Rosario and Schrimshaw 2013; Mustanski, Chivers and Bailey 2002). Sexual identity, though generally stable for most individuals, is for others fluid over time, particularly among adolescents and women (Mock and Eibach 2012; Mustanski, Kuper and Greene 2013; Diamond 2008). It is better, then, for both clinicians and religious communities to walk alongside people like Nate with epistemological and moral humility, providing support and care in the context of deeply personal journeys without subsuming them into any preexisting cultural scripts.

References

APA (2009) *Report of the American Psychological Association Task Force on Appropriate Therapeutic Responses to Sexual Orientation*. Washington, DC: American Psychological Association.

Diamond, L.M. (2008) *Sexual Fluidity: Understanding Women's Love and Desire*. Cambridge, MA: Harvard University Press.

Mock, S.E. and Eibach, R.P. (2012) 'Stability and change in sexual orientation identity over a 10-year period in adulthood.' *Archives of Sexual Behavior 41*, 3, 641–648.

Mustanski, B.S., Chivers, M.L. and Bailey, J.M. (2002) 'A critical review of recent biological research on human sexual orientation.' *Annual Review of Sex Research* *13*, 1, 89–140.

Mustanski, B., Kuper, L. and Greene, G.J. (2013) 'Development of sexual orientation and identity.' In D.L. Tolman and L.M. Diamond (eds) *APA Handbook of Sexuality and Psychology, Volume 1*. Washington, DC: American Psychological Association, 597–628.

Rosario, M. and Schrimshaw, E.W. (2013) 'Theories and etiologies of sexual orientation.' In D.L. Tolman and L.M. Diamond (eds) *APA Handbook of Sexuality and Psychology, Volume 1*. Washington, DC: American Psychological Association, 555–596.

Part 3
Palliative Case Studies

Steve Nolan

Spiritual care has an acknowledged place within palliative care. Care of the dying has historically been a religious duty, and the founding mothers of what has become the Hospice Movement were deeply religious people: Mme Jeanne Garnier (Lyon, France, 1842); Sister Mary Augustine (Dublin, 1879, and Hackney, London, 1905); Mother Alphonsa (New York, 1899); and Dame Cicely Saunders (Sydenham, London, 1967, the first 'modern' hospice) (Clark 1999, 2012). However, the centrality of that place is becoming less certain over time, as palliative care becomes increasingly a medical specialty and as the economic model becomes increasingly dominant within healthcare. The cases presented here, none of which come from a hospice setting, demonstrate the value of good spiritual care for the dying.

The work presented by Chaplains Huth and Roberts draws attention to the religious aspect of spiritual care. As a lifelong Roman Catholic, the 91-year-old veteran, Andrew, living with vascular dementia and prostate cancer, was strengthened by regular contact with the religious rituals 'of his life's faith practice'. This included attending Mass, but he also found strength in praying the Lord's Prayer with his evangelical protestant chaplain. Andrew's spiritual care underscores the fact that the sacraments are an important aspect of care for many Christians, and indexes the value of both religious ritual and, by extension, any familiar ritual for those who are dying. The spiritual value of the sacramental ritual is not diminished by terming it 'cognitive support'. Norman Autton, the Anglican chaplain claimed as the father of modern British chaplaincy (Swift 2009, p.45), argued that the chaplain should 'exercise his (*sic*) sacramental ministry' with 'sensitive concern' as 'an important part of his whole expression of caring' (Autton 1968, p.46). But Autton warned against the impersonal distribution of sacraments:

> It is as easy for [the priest/chaplain] to hide behind the ritual of the sacraments as it is for the doctor to remain impersonal behind his (*sic*) mask or stethoscope. He (*sic*) can minister the sacraments frequently, and yet at the same time remain aloof from any meaningful relationship or genuine 'I–Thou' encounter with the patient. (Autton 1966, p.76)

The interaction between Chaplain Roberts and Andrew models the tenderness and compassion – the love – that transforms mere ritual into authentic spiritual care.

Listening is a core skill all chaplains must develop. Autton (1966) distinguished between *passive listening*, 'which can be used when stress is great, and the dying one anxious to talk about his fear and frustrations' (Autton 1966, p.61), and *active or directed listening*, 'which perhaps calls for even greater skill, and is coupled with the art of asking questions and so encouraging the patient to talk' (Autton 1966, p.61). In his work with Lee, Andrew's daughter, Chaplain Huth demonstrates the skill with real subtlety, preferring to call it *deep listening* – what some counsellors/therapists call *advanced empathy*. This is the skill of attending to 'what is present in a person that has not yet been spoken', picking up on the hints that a person is giving about themselves, which they themselves are missing in their own narrative. A good example is where Lee is trying to make sense of her father's suffering: essentially asking why bad things happen to good people, she slips in her thought that things 'would be so different for him now'. Sensitive to the importance of what Lee had missed, Chaplain Huth paraphrases her words and asks a question that leads Lee, perhaps unexpectedly, to realize the pride her father felt towards her.

Lee had requested to speak with Chaplain Huth, but chaplains in palliative care are frequently proactive, seeking to build supportive relationships with people who would not otherwise engage with a religious person. In Chaplain Redl's case, David, an Orthodox Jewish inhabitant of Old Jerusalem, had rejected his religious community and his God, and had no use for a religious figure, such as a chaplain. His life experiences of loss and abandonment had left him emotionally both isolated from, and insulated against, close human relationships; and Chaplain Redl's initial, and perhaps naïve, offer of support was dismissed abruptly. Her subsequent work with David is an example of how, through gentle patience, a chaplain might earn the right to speak. Knowing little, if anything, of his life story, Chaplain Redl quickly realizes that words alone would not be the right medium with which to create a safe space for David, and instead takes the risk of offering her presence and some unobtrusive acts of kindness, with the intention of communicating: 'I am there…[and] I can wait until you are ready to reach out.' Her intuitive approach resists the temptation to go deeper, and so get ahead of David; instead, she calculates the risk of alienating him, and having him 'close up again', against the risk of not helping him in the way she felt she best could. In the end, Chaplain Redl's careful approach is vindicated when, gradually, David takes his own risk and reveals his story of abandonment and loneliness.

What is striking about the relationship Chaplain Redl creates with David is that its quality could have been measured in his reduced need for pain relief. The point Chaplain Redl makes is that a considerable amount of David's physical pain was existential, resulting not just from his cancer but from 'his sense of abandonment by his family and God, his loneliness and lack of purpose'. The phenomenon Chaplain Redl describes is frequently identified in palliative care as 'total pain', a term coined by Cicely Saunders. The term has value in that it acknowledges that suffering can be a complex of contributing factors (physical, psychological/emotional, social and spiritual, categories whose boundaries are arbitrary and negotiable); however, in clinical practice its use adds little beyond the use of terms like 'spiritual or existential pain or distress'. Chaplain Redl does not use the term 'total pain' but identifies that David's distress is rooted in his feelings of abandonment and loneliness. In addressing these feelings through her companionship, Chaplain Redl shows how it is possible for spiritual care to bring about some measurable degree of relief.

The final case offers an extraordinary insight into the culture and sacred practices of a Native American family and an example of how the chaplain can be an invaluable resource to both the institution and the family. The degree of cultural difference managed by Chaplain Weyls in the case he presents is daunting. The case centres around Esmeralda, an 85-year-old Native American woman, and her culturally Native and religiously Catholic family. Esmeralda's family needed to celebrate both their traditional Native American death rituals and the 'last rites' of the Roman Catholic Church. Chaplain Weyls, a Caucasian male of mostly European descent, had been an ordained Roman Catholic priest, but at the time of the case he was in the process of having his priestly ordination recognized by the Episcopal Church. Besides supporting Esmeralda's family, Chaplain Weyls saw his task as serving as host and facilitator for holy men of two traditions: Robert, a Native American Holy Man of the Crow tribe; and Fr Alois, a Roman Catholic priest and native Tanzanian of the Chagga people. In this situation, Chaplain Weyls shows how, when the chaplain humbly adopts the attitude of a willing student, rather than the spiritual expert, it is possible to represent and resource the institution while advocating for and supporting the family.

In presenting his case, Chaplain Weyls focuses a question that all chaplains must at some point address to themselves: What approach to spiritual care will allow me, with integrity, to claim my own faith perspective while at the same time be open to the spiritual experiences and values of others? This is a question vital to good spiritual care practice, which, as in this case, is increasingly delivered in secular institutions and which, therefore, is delivered to all people, regardless of religious affiliation or lack thereof. Chaplain Weyls has answered this question to his own satisfaction and has developed what he calls his 'operative theology of spiritual care'. His theology is 'fundamentally Christian, sacramental and incarnational', and it enables him to serve and support people of differing spiritual and religious beliefs without threatening the integrity of his own faith understanding.

In responding to these cases, David Mitchell identifies a number of themes the cases illustrate. Co-author of the 'Spiritual and religious care competencies for specialist palliative care' (Marie Curie Cancer Care 2003), he writes as a Scottish chaplain and draws particular attention to the central importance of self-awareness for all chaplains, and he connects this with the chaplain's rootedness in a community of faith (or in the case of a humanist chaplain, belief). Mitchell underlines the need for chaplains to see themselves as part of the multidisciplinary team and makes a timely point about how essential it is that chaplains keep up to date with current thinking in spiritual care.

The final response from Barbara Pesut, a Canadian nurse researcher, is informed by the perspective of one who understands that chaplains are frequently invisible within the healthcare system. She observes that chaplains in general, but palliative care chaplains in particular, work in the liminal spaces, waiting there with those for whom they care. Pesut notes the way the chaplains in this section offer care that is directed at sustaining personhood at the end of life. She specifically mentions dementia, and the value of familiar rituals and prayers in spiritual care. And with reference to Chaplain Huth's work with Lee, she highlights the importance of religious ethics as an aspect of care often neglected by other healthcare professionals. In this context, Pesut coins the term 'religious and spiritual navigator' as a new metaphor for the chaplain who is competent to negotiate the religious and spiritual plurality of modern healthcare.

References

Autton, N. (1966) *The Pastoral Care of the Dying (The Library of Pastoral Care)*. London: SPCK.

Autton, N. (1968) *Pastoral Care in Hospitals (The Library of Pastoral Care)*. London: SPCK.

Clark, D. (1999) 'Cradled to the grave? Terminal care in the United Kingdom, 1948–67.' *Mortality* 4, 3, 225–247.

Clark, D. (2012) 'Hospice in historical perspective.' Available at www.deathreference. com/Ho-Ka/Hospice-in-Historical-Perspective.html#b, accessed on 4 July 2014.

Marie Curie Cancer Care (2003) 'Spiritual and religious care competencies for specialist palliative care.' Available at www.mariecurie.org.uk/Documents/healthcare-professionals/spritual-religious-care-competencies.pdf, accessed on 4 July 2014.

Swift, C. (2009) *Hospital Chaplaincy in the Twenty-first Century: The Crisis of Spiritual Care on the NHS*. Farnham, VT: Ashgate Publishing.

Chapter 11
'I need to do the right thing for him'

– Andrew, a Canadian veteran at the
end of his life, and his daughter Lee

Jim Huth and Wes Roberts

Introduction

This case study illustrates the end-of-life spiritual care interventions, and their outcomes, of two chaplains at the Sunnybrook Veterans Centre, a long-term care facility at Sunnybrook Health Sciences Centre. The interventions employed are referenced to concepts that have been described recently in the literature.

Sunnybrook has a long and proud tradition of caring for Canada's war veterans. It is the largest veterans care facility in Canada and offers long-term and complex continuing care to 500 veterans from the Second World War (WWII) and the Korean War. Veteran residents live as independently as possible within a supportive environment. The facility provides cognitive support, physical support, mental health, stroke and palliative care for veterans. Almost half of the residents at the Centre suffer from Alzheimer's disease and other dementias.

The case is about Andrew, a 91-year-old veteran diagnosed with vascular dementia and carcinoma of the prostate, and his daughter, Lee. Andrew's identified spiritual needs were to maintain the personal dimension of his life's faith practice, including attending religious services, having prayer and spiritual companionship and to spend time in the facility's therapeutic garden. Lee's stated spiritual need was to address feelings of isolation due to carrying the weight of her father's care by herself. She also expressed feelings of confusion and ambivalence about how best to address her father's palliative care status with his healthcare team, especially with his physician.

Andrew had been a respected training officer in the Royal Canadian Air Force (RCAF) during WWII, after which he had a successful career in the pulp and paper industry until his retirement. Andrew was a widower to his late wife, Barbara, after 60 years of marriage. She died a few months prior to his admission to the Veterans Centre. Both his children, Lee and Ed, are in their mid-fifties. Lee is married with one son; Ed is divorced and has two children. Andrew named Lee as his healthcare substitute decision maker (SDM). She was his primary support person. Andrew was raised Roman Catholic and had found it to be a source of comfort and support throughout his life. He and his wife raised their children in the same faith.

The chaplains in this case study are middle-aged and work full-time at Sunnybrook. Wes is ordained in an evangelical tradition and has worked at the Veterans Centre for 10 years. He has advanced standing with the Canadian Association for Spiritual Care (CASC). Jim is a Roman Catholic priest and has been with the Veterans Centre for 3 years. He has over 25 years' experience as a spiritual care provider and is a certified specialist with CASC. Wes's involvement with Andrew and his daughter took place over an 8-year period. Jim's involvement was limited to a few months prior to Andrew's death and was based on Lee's request for Roman Catholic rituals for her father and spiritual support for herself.

Due to the lengthy history of the spiritual care relationship, and in order to highlight specific spiritual needs, interventions and outcomes that seemed beneficial to Andrew and Lee, the case study limits discussion to pivotal meetings at the end of Andrew's life.

The study is an anonymized version of actual spiritual care encounters. We have permission from the administration of the Veterans Centre and Sunnybrook Health Sciences Centre to publish this case study. We received written consent from Andrew's daughter to write the case study based on our work with her and her father.

Case study

History of the spiritual care relationships with Wes

Andrew lived for 8 years on one of the cognitive support units where I (Wes) am assigned. During this period, his various spiritual needs were addressed primarily through one-to-one contact with me and via the weekly on-unit worship service structured for persons with advanced dementia. These services emphasized that all persons – even those with cognitive impairment – are spiritual beings, still capable of having a unique relationship with God (Kneller 1971). At the conclusion of many of these services, Andrew would tell me, 'Oh, I feel very good'. During his final months, an essential aspect of my spiritual care intervention was to assist Andrew in addressing his need to feel spiritually connected and not isolated at the end of life and, because of the progression of his dementia, to provide him with spiritual companionship related to his feeling of being 'closed-in and lost'. Due to Andrew's physical decline, interventions occurred through a series of bedside visits intended to maintain continuity of care and therapeutic support.

Visit with Andrew

One particular afternoon, Andrew was alert and in a bright mood and responded spontaneously when engaged.

> *Wes:* Good afternoon, Andrew. (*pause*) It's Wes, the chaplain. (*pause*) I was thinking about you today.

Andrew: (pause) Oh boy, that's nice. *(Chuckles and smiles.)*

Wes: (Moving closer to the bedrail, speaking in a slow, measured tone.) How is life treating you today?

Andrew: I have had a good day, but I slept most of it away. *(chuckles)*

Wes: I believe sleep is an important thing. *(pause)* I'm curious, Andrew, what is making today so good?

Andrew: I spent time praying.

Wes: What I have learned about you is that prayer is important for you.

I was affirming his practice of prayer as a source of meaning; Andrew was nodding his head slowly.

Wes: Would you find a prayer meaningful to you right now?

Andrew: (Nodding again.) I sure would.

I offered to pray the Lord's Prayer with Andrew, which I have used with him as a cognitive orientation strategy. I recited it slowly and with measure. Andrew spontaneously entered in while maintaining eye contact with me.

Andrew and Wes in unison: …forever and ever. Amen.

Andrew: (unsolicited) Oh boy, that was nice. *(A large grin came to his face and he laughed.)*

Wes: Yes, I would agree. *(pause)* Andrew, how are you feeling right now?

Andrew: Oh…so peaceful.

In the weeks that followed, my visits became increasingly less verbal and began to embody a vigil of supportive presence at his bedside.

Subsequent visit with Andrew

Two weeks later, I visited Andrew at bedside. He appeared drowsy.

Wes: Hi, Andrew. It's Wes, the chaplain, to see you.

Andrew slowly opened his eyes. He acknowledged me with a nod. After a brief pause, Andrew offered words that were indiscernible. I prompted him to repeat what he was attempting to communicate.

Andrew: (*Whispered tone.*) I feel closer.

Wes: Closer to whom, Andrew?

Andrew: Closer to my father.

Wes: Do you mean closer to your 'Father' God?

Nodding his head when he heard the term 'Father God', Andrew closed his eyes. He made no further verbal response. I then affirmed Andrew's expression of closeness.

Wes: Thank you, Andrew, may you enjoy the feeling of closeness with God.

I maintained companionship at his bedside with a vigil presence.

Over the years of providing spiritual care to Andrew, I have also spent time with Lee to provide grief support surrounding the unexpected death of her mother. During those visits, I supported her in the fears she had of losing her father in a similar manner. When changes in Andrew's health arose, Lee would become anxious and fearful that he would not recover. She constantly consulted the medical team to determine the causes of these changes. As Andrew's health declined, Lee said she wanted 'to do the right thing'.

History of the spiritual care relationships with Jim

Wes asked me (Jim) to contact Lee because she wanted to speak with a priest to ensure that she was doing 'the right thing'. She wanted Andrew to have the Sacrament of the Sick. Moreover, Wes told me that Lee had a strong need to talk, feeling only someone from her own faith tradition could give her the answers she needed for the questions she was raising.

The first time Lee and I spoke was by telephone. She requested to Wes that I call her first, preferring initially not to meet face to face.

First contact with Lee

When I identified myself, I sensed tentativeness in her voice. She told me that she was nervous about talking to a priest. She felt she could not be herself and was concerned about 'how things might come out in their presence'. I assured her that, like Wes, I was a trained chaplain and that my role was to provide spiritual care and counselling to veterans and their families. I invited her to be herself and to speak in a way that was comfortable to her. I listened to her in a reflective and non-judgemental way, and in the process she told her story – one that she grappled with emotionally and spiritually.

The conversation helped Lee to share the burdens that she had been carrying as her father's primary caregiver when he was living at home. Her father was all-important to her, the one person in her life who 'Truly understood me when I was growing up. I always felt so much closer to my dad than to my mother.' Lee told me that her mother died shortly before her father was admitted to the Veterans Centre. 'Mother didn't linger like my father is now.' She also spoke of her frustration with her brother's lack of involvement. Now that her father's health was rapidly declining in the Veterans Centre, Ed had left her with making all the healthcare decisions. According to her, Ed offered little input, leaving her to wonder if she was making the 'right decisions'.

Lee was a highly successful executive in advertising and had close relationships with her husband, son and two women who were lifelong friends. Nevertheless, she spoke from a place of deep isolation. Lee also expressed a sense of pride and strength in her resolve to help her father at this last stage of his life. In addition, she expressed surprise in being able to talk candidly with me. Although the original purpose of the telephone call was to address her queries about rituals for her father, it was clear that Lee first needed to speak from her heart of how her father's physical decline was impacting her and of the emotional challenges she was facing in being his SDM. Lee ended the conversation by letting me know that, although not a practising Roman Catholic, she turned to her faith during times of difficulty. 'My father taught me to rely on faith to get you through troubles. He did, especially during the war.'

Lee asked if we could talk again, and I gave her my contact information at the hospital. As consistency of care was essential to supporting Lee spiritually, both ethically and from a professional practice perspective, I explained that it would be helpful for Wes to know that Lee wanted to see me again to address further her spiritual needs. I reinforced that the care that I would be providing was not to duplicate or interfere with the work that Wes had given Lee and she gave me permission to inform Wes of the salient points of our conversation.

Second contact with Lee

A week later, Lee came to my office after visiting her father. I invited her to sit down and she immediately began speaking.

Lee: I was visiting my father. The nurse was giving him his medications, so I thought I would come to your office. Is this a good time for you?

Jim: Yes, it is. How's your father?

Lee: Not too well. He's agitated. The nurse said he had a difficult night. He couldn't sleep. I keep wondering if he is trying to tell me something.

Jim: It sounds like you are feeling that he has something on his mind that will not let go of him.

Lee: With his dementia, I am not sure what he's saying makes sense. He was always so strong and had a great mind. I don't understand why it has to be like this. I thought it would be so different for him now. He's a good man, a wonderful father. He served in the war.

Jim: You seem to have a strong sense of how your father's life would be now. Yet, his life now seems like a contradiction of what you envisioned. Lee, how did you envision his life to be now?

Lee: He would be home with me. He would be listening to classical music, working in the garden, talking and laughing with me.

Jim: What would he be saying to you?

Lee: He would ask me how my day went; ask me what my son and husband were up to. He'd tell me how much he loved all of us. My father would say, 'Be more understanding of your brother; we don't know what made him move away from us. We don't know what it's like to be him; we just know how frustrating it is for us not being able to change him.'

Jim: Anything else?

Lee: No matter what we would be talking about – the good or bad – he would always end with saying how proud he has been of me.

I could have responded by picking up on Lee's relationship with her brother. Instead, I decided to stay with the central figure of her story.

Jim: Tell me what it means when you say that your father is proud of you.

She took her time. Her eyes began to water up. She took a tissue from her purse.

Lee: Proud means that he believes in me; he sees beyond my mistakes. He sees what I have done in my life. I was a hippie growing up. He supported me always. No matter what anyone else thought of me, I turned my life around. I have a wonderful husband and son, and I'm successful in my business.

Jim: It sounds like being proud allows you to stand confidently in your father's belief and love for you. How are you proud of him, especially at this time of his life?

Lee: I'm proud of his service during the war, his work ethic, being able to still smile at me when I walk in his room now – the smile that he always smiled. I'm amazed that he still has faith in God even when his body is breaking down. It's getting difficult for him to eat. Yet, he told me that if he ever got like this, he would be OK.

Jim: What do you think OK would look like for him?

Lee: He would be ready to take that final step that is needed to let go. He said his faith in God would bring him not only to Heaven, but also to my mother. And that I would be OK after he's gone.

Jim: Lee, who would be most surprised to hear you talk this way, expressing confidently what you're proud of about your dad, especially his faith that helps him take his final step?

Lee: My mother. (*I asked why.*) Because she and I would have our share of disagreements, especially about his health. Being responsible would surprise her. Yet, in some ways, she wouldn't be that surprised, because like my father, I knew she had faith in me. I think she would be proud of me too.

Jim: How did she have faith in you?

Lee: When I did crazy things, she would shake her head, tell me to be more serious and then put her arms lovingly around me. This made all the difference.

Jim: How do you think your father's faith might be helping him now, especially as you connect it with your mother?

Lee: It is helping him to trust that God will see him through this – give him a peaceful death when it is his time. My mother believed that too for herself.

Jim: Since he trusts you would be OK when his health is declining, how does being OK show up for you in your life right now?

Lee: Things which are OK for me? I know that his nurses are doing their best. I am driving his doctor crazy with my questions – but I have to know. Finding a priest to help my father have his sacraments is making it OK, and knowing that you and Wes are listening to me. What is not OK is I'm losing my father; I'll never see him again.

Jim: There is nothing that feels OK about that.

Lee: I hate this time now. It is breaking my heart. I feel powerless. I want him better, but seeing him, I know that's not going to happen.

She cried from the depths of her pain. I sat silently, not interrupting her from getting in touch with her pain and its source.

Lee: I just want him to be at peace – that's why I want you to meet him. At least I can do that for him.

Jim: I will see him.

Lee: He likes the Lord's Prayer. He prayed it during the war to get him through. You have to say it slowly so he can say it with you. I also want to talk with you about the last rites – is it still called that? I am not ready for that yet, but I know I will be, because that is what he wants.

Jim: I am able to see him today. I'll see if he would like to pray the Lord's Prayer together. We can talk later about administering the Anointing of the Sick, which it is called now.

Lee: It is time for me to get back to my father. I will tell him that you will visit him. Did it surprise you that I was a hippie? (*We both laughed.*)

Jim: Why do I get the feeling that you were the first hippie in Canada?

Lee: My father thought I was. He said I was always high-spirited. I would say or do what I wanted, but cautious that, when all was said and done, I needed to be sensible. I guess that whoever I was, my father was always proud of me. Thanks for talking with me. I would like to talk again.

Jim: That sounds good. Let me know.

First visit with Andrew

Upon arriving on the unit, Andrew's nurse informed me that he appeared slightly anxious. When I entered his room, which he shared with two other veterans, Andrew was sitting in his wheelchair. On the wall near his bed were pictures of Andrew and his family at different times of his life; one of Andrew in his RCAF uniform portrayed a youthful, strong and confident man. Age and time took away his vigour, strength and his health, but not his smile; it was that same smile that he had as I entered his room. When I began to speak to him, his smile faded; he became slightly agitated. He did not respond verbally when I engaged him. When I let him know that his daughter asked me to visit him, his agitation seemed to decrease slightly. I then asked if he would like to say the Lord's Prayer with me. He consented with a nod. As I began the prayer, he mouthed it with me. Afterwards, his agitation seemed to have decreased more. I said goodbye to him and let him know I would return. I conferred with his nurse about his decreased agitation and documented the visit.

Third contact with Lee

Prior to our third meeting, Andrew's healthcare team had informed Lee about his rapid physical decline. When we met, Lee expressed a sense of ambivalence about his being on comfort measures, and about her meeting with the team, as illustrated in the following dialogue.

Lee: (With tears in her eyes.) By letting him go, does that mean I am letting him down? Am I abandoning him?

Jim: I am not sure I understand what you are asking. What did the healthcare team tell you?

Lee: It won't be long now. He is not responding. The focus is on comfort and I am thinking we need to try something else to give him another chance. I don't want him to think that I am giving up on him.

Jim: Giving up? Is that what you mean by not wanting to abandon him?

Lee: Yes, that's exactly what it means!

Jim: Tell me about not wanting to abandon him.

Lee: That I am not going to leave him like this.

I asked her to help me understand what 'like this' means.

> *Lee:* It means that he really is dying. I don't want him to die. I know comfort care is what he wants. My family, people here told me I have to prepare myself for this day, but no matter how much I try to prepare, I can never be ready for this. I can't abandon him to death. What am I supposed to do?

> *Jim:* I can't tell you what to do, but maybe if you feel that you are supposed to do something – does this go back to your feeling the need to do the 'right thing' for your father? (*She nodded.*) Where does this feeling come from?

> *Lee:* Whenever he had to make tough choices, he always seemed to do the right thing.

> *Jim:* Now the tough choice is on you. (*She nodded.*) When you're facing difficult situations, to whom do you usually turn?

> *Lee:* Right now I am thinking only of my father.

> *Jim:* What would he be saying to you?

> *Lee:* (*laughing*) He would be asking me, 'Lee, when were you so concerned about doing the right thing? You always did your own thing, and if you didn't know what to do, you would come to me.'

> *Jim:* So, what does that mean to you?

> *Lee:* Maybe, my father wasn't as caught up with me doing the right thing as much as he was making sure that I didn't have to face things alone. After all, I found myself in some real messes, and he said that we would get through it.

> *Jim:* Does now feel like one of those times – like a mess? (*She nodded.*) Then what do you envision your father saying with respect to getting through this?

> *Lee:* He told me he couldn't live forever – he didn't want to. He told me that, when it was his time, to let him go. But I don't know if this is the time.

Jim: How would your father respond to that?

Lee: I don't know.

Jim: Would it help to consider what the healthcare team said about your father's present condition?

She agreed and reviewed what was said to her about her father's rapid decline. This review allowed her to decide for herself that she had not left 'any stone unturned'.

Lee: I keep thinking of what he's been telling me: 'I will be with your mother again.'

Jim: When you hear that, what is it saying to you?

Lee: As much as I hate to admit it, maybe it's staying the course.

I asked what that course might be.

Lee: It's comfort measures.

Jim: Lee, when you hear your father's words, 'I will be with your mother again', what does that say to you?

Lee: It makes me think that if he is ready to leave, then I have to think about my readiness to let him go.

Jim: Do you have a sense of that readiness?

Lee: I was thinking of what he said: 'When it's time for me to go – let me go.' He believes he will be OK. Why do I feel that he believes I will be OK too?

Jim: From that question, I am sensing you feel that your father knows you pretty well.

She concluded our visit stating, 'I know that his love for me doesn't die. I'll always have that.'

Joint contact with Andrew and Lee

After our third contact, Lee asked me to administer the sacrament of the Anointing of the Sick to her father. I explained that the sacrament is not confined to those who are about to die, and that the spiritual practice of the sacrament includes having loved ones gather to support the sick person with prayer, readings and rituals, including holy oil. Lee told me she wanted to be present for it, and asked if Wes and some of Andrew's nurses could participate. She also wanted to invite her brother, Ed. Lee felt that now the two of them ought to come together to pray for their father. At Lee's invitation, he agreed to be a part of the sacrament.

After I anointed Andrew, I invited Lee, Ed, Wes and the nurses, if they wished, to speak of what stood out for each of them about Andrew. This allowed them to be active participants in the sacrament and to speak openly, not only for Andrew to hear their words to strengthen him in the grace of the sacrament, but also to comfort *them*. Lee and Ed spoke their words of gratefulness and devotion for their father, and of how they loved him. Afterwards, Lee commented, 'When you anointed him, my father looked so peaceful. I knew that whatever happens, he would be all right. In seeing this, I am feeling peace.'

Discussion

The importance of spiritual care as an essential component of palliative care has been universally recognized and accepted since the start of the hospice moment in the 1960s, and is reinforced in the World Health Organization's definition of palliative care (WHO 2002). McClain, Rosenfeld and Breitbart (2003) found that spiritual well-being seems to guard against end-of-life despair. Their study suggests that spirituality-based interventions may be useful in helping terminally ill persons find peace and meaning. Spirituality has been found to be an important predictor of improving the quality of life of persons receiving palliative care (Hermann 2001; McClain *et al.* 2003). A literature review by Dein and Stygall (1997) highlights that, from a coping perspective, religion can reduce the psychological morbidity associated with chronic illness and terminal illness. Palliative care chaplains have a distinct position on healthcare teams as being active and deep listeners to the spiritual distress of patients and their families. Deep listening involves more than rephrasing, reframing and acknowledging what is heard. Deep listening pays attention to what is present in a person that has not yet been spoken. In listening deeply to a person's narrative, chaplains help the person move from 'the known and the familiar' to 'what is possible to know' (White 2007, p.277; Russell and Carey 2004, pp.23–24).

In terms of family perspectives on dying, Wilson and Daley (1999) found that providing spiritual support was important to families, especially support which included staff talking about religious and spiritual matters, as well as offering prayers and visits from clergy. Thus, a regular review of spiritual needs of the patient and family ought to guide the practice of the chaplain. Such a review can ensure that spiritual care is flexible and adaptable (Hermann 2001; Wilson and Daley 1999), particularly when those needs change.

Less commonly spoken of, when addressing the provision of spiritual care in palliative care, is the impact of dementia, and how the spirituality of an older person needs to be cared for and understood. Bell and Troxel (2001) identify eight spiritual needs of persons living with dementia: to feel connected; to be respected and appreciated; to be loved; to be known and accepted; to be compassionate; to give and to share; to be productive and successful; and to have hope. In reference to these authors, Smith (2005) comments that, in light of the debilitating nature of dementia, an obvious challenge facing chaplains is to appreciate, for example, what it means for a person with dementia to achieve success and to understand how this is measured for the person. Smith notes that what is most important in such an example, and in the overall care of the person, is the emphasis on simplicity: to recognize a simple need and fulfil it can in itself be viewed as successful (Smith 2005, p.14). In attending to this need for simplicity, the chaplain's unique role is one of spiritual companionship, including, if possible, helping the person find a way to express what is meaningful to them. This is the type of role that we attempted to have with Andrew.

Assessment, interventions and outcomes
ANDREW

After serving with distinction in the RCAF, Andrew married Barbara, the love of his life, and together they raised their two children. Lee's high-spirited nature at times exasperated her mother and caused some stress between them. In later years, the emotional distance that Ed put between himself and the rest of the family served as a source of tension among them. In spite of such challenges, Andrew looked for ways to inspire his family and find ways to remain close. This search was built on his lifelong faith in God and his boundless love for his family.

Shamy (2003) asserts that providing spiritual care to persons near death – especially to those with declining mental powers – is often a work done in a wilderness of loss. What is needed is a path through the wilderness which endows the dying person with value, respect and integrity, and where they can find reconciliation. As he approached his death, Andrew seemed to experience that sense of being in the wilderness. In an endeavour to create a path with Andrew, Wes sought to understand what his word 'father' meant for Andrew at this moment in his life.

Each encounter that we had with Andrew mirrored Smith's principle of responding to a person's spiritual needs through the simplicity of companionship (Smith 2005). First, Andrew's practice of praying the Lord's Prayer provided the opportunity to facilitate and affirm his profession of inward peace, even with an advanced dementia diagnosis and facing the end of life. The value of prayer remained present to him during times of feeling 'closed-in and lost'. Through attentive spiritual companionship and the use of familiar prayer intervention, Wes enabled Andrew to feel supported in his connectedness with God. This was especially the case when he participated in worship. Considering

Kneller's personal idealist approach towards reality, the worship services' premise acknowledges that God transcends all impairment (Kneller 1971). Using therapeutic techniques, including time and space orientation, name repetition, memory cueing and the use of familiar hymns within a basic liturgical form, the worship service that Wes led acknowledged the physical world that Andrew shared with other cognitively impaired persons who attended the service.

By active companionship, Wes witnessed Andrew's expression of feeling closer to the Sacred – possibly another way for Andrew to claim control over death and feel peaceful, which can be an existential expression of a lifetime's devotion to his faith. At significant moments throughout the progression of his dementia, we gave priority to Andrew expressing his spiritual needs, especially praying with him and giving him the anointing sacrament. This sacrament provided him with a sense of the Divine and the acknowledged love of his family, which seemed to comfort him. These interventions and outcomes helped his healthcare team to appreciate his spiritual needs being satisfied, which impacted positively on his overall care, especially as he approached death. The impact of attending to these needs helped empower Andrew to claim his sources of meaning at the closing of his life.

Following Andrew's death, the final expression of spiritual companionship to him was for chaplaincy to conduct a bedside flag ceremony – a civilian, non-religious tribute offered to Sunnybrook veterans to honour their life and their veteran heritage. This ceremony, developed by Wes, allows assembled family and healthcare team members the opportunity to express their feelings and the option to share significant memories of the veteran's life. The closing of the ceremony involves the communal draping of a Canadian flag over the veteran's body. This act of remembrance evokes a time of comfort, affirmation and peace.

LEE

Before her mother died, Lee had focused substantially on being her caregiver. After her death, the bond between Lee and her father intensified as she devoted herself to his care. In this role, she attempted to care for him in ways that reflected his care for her throughout her life. In reciprocation, she was his faithful advocate. In this role, however, she felt isolated in being the decision maker in her father's medical care.

Lee received a number of spiritual care interventions, the outcomes of which proved beneficial to the relief of her feeling isolated. She experienced us as spiritual companions who helped her name the burdens she carried as primary caregiver, as well as to address what was most difficult for her and to find ways through those difficulties. She discovered that faith in herself, and in its various expressions, could serve her well in being her father's SDM. Moreover, she asserted a sense of pride and strength in her determination to support her father at the end of his life.

Lee did not identify herself as religious but nevertheless felt an affinity to the faith of her parents. She sought religious support for her father and spiritual care for herself, despite her discomfort with religious authority. Chaplaincy used active listening and unconditional positive regard as Lee spoke of her uneasiness when talking to persons in religious authority. She expressed ease in being able to speak her truth with Jim. When Jim invited her to be herself and speak in a way which was comfortable to her, Lee was helped to feel valued and to appreciate that what she said mattered. Lee expressed gratitude to us both for our spiritual support, indicating she trusted us to listen deeply to her spiritual struggle.

Due to her strong emotional attachment to her father, Lee's spiritual struggle was to understand how faith and trust could see her through the devastating anguish of losing him. Our role as chaplains was not to contest or mould the ways she articulated her religious values and spiritual reflections, but to listen deeply to her distress and help her find ways to frame her spiritual identity, and so find some degree of peace in letting Andrew go.

Lee knew she could not easily let go of her feelings of hurt towards her brother's decision to have little involvement with the family. Nevertheless, she felt it was important for Ed to be part of the sacrament for her father. In particular, what stood out for her in the most recent weeks was that her brother had visited Andrew. Lee expressed that seeing Ed connecting with their father enabled her to be more willing to speak to Ed about the hurt she felt in their relationship. She sensed from Ed's willingness to listen that he was trying to be more caring towards her. By participating in the sacrament, Lee and Ed seemed liberated to say in each other's presence what they each needed to say to their father; they spoke without inhibition of the meaningful family memories they shared and of what they both valued and loved about their father. In this way, spiritual counselling and support gave access to a ritual that offered comfort and meaning to Andrew's family (Orchard and Clark 2001). We sensed Lee's hope that being together with their father would help her and Ed to be together for one another in their father's remaining days, and perhaps even afterwards.

In terms of her mother, Lee was able to let go of concentrating on the things that they disagreed about, and to name what bonded them together as mother and daughter – the faith her mother had in Lee. This enabled Lee to acknowledge that her mother, like her father, would be proud of her. An intervention Jim used was to invite Lee to consider who would be surprised to hear her speak with confidence about how she was committed to caring for her father. Responding that her mother would be surprised reminded Lee of valued times and feelings in their relationship, and perhaps helped her feel less alone in tending to her father, and so reclaim her own spirit of authority and discover its blessings and strength.

Lee needed to speak at length about the things she found most troubling and overwhelming: how to be with her father and support him in his dying. Lee's preferred way of making sense of these things was to speak of them through stories. Jim used deep listening to engage her in the cherished stories she told. This was especially the case in attending to the words she used to tell her story and how these stories intersected with one another. How people use and define words are important to the way they see their situation and themselves; words are also important in helping people see new possibilities of how to face those situations (White 2007; Russell and Carey 2004). Attending to Lee's words ('proud', 'OK', 'trust', 'faith') gave opportunities to explore more deeply how she understood them. Such conversations allowed rich descriptions of these words, making them more meaningful to Lee and more relevant in helping to address her spiritual needs and the overall care of her father. Deep listening was used as an intervention to help Lee envision her story as one that was not overshadowed by her ambivalence about Andrew being on comfort measures, as illustrated in Jim's third contact. Specifically, Lee was empowered to speak of the intensity of what it meant to lose her father and his acceptance of his impending death. She became more accepting of herself in how she handled her father's care, and opened herself to a relationship with her father that transcended death: 'I know that his love for me doesn't die.'

When Lee cried as she felt the agony of never seeing her father again, Jim offered her a spiritual care presence of 'sitting with her' in the pain of her grief, since no intervening words could ease her immeasurable pain. The hope was that this facilitated silence would indicate to her that her agony, and how she expressed it, would not be dismissed or minimized, but rather valued. The intervention of 'sitting with her' helped Lee to be uninhibited in speaking of the effect her father's death would have on her. As part of addressing the challenge 'to let go', Jim invited Lee to reflect on what would be the 'right thing' to do and to review how she understood Andrew's health status. This review enabled Lee to determine for herself that she had done all she could for her father. Thus, she felt empowered to tend to him in ways that allowed her to reciprocate in the manner he had always tended to her: with a sense of profound love and gratitude.

Conclusion

This was a complex case involving multilayered and intersecting storylines, which influenced how Lee, in particular, addressed her father's end-of-life care. This was especially demonstrated in Jim's second contact with Lee. Jim recognized that he could have addressed any one of the intersecting themes that she raised in terms of how she felt towards her brother, mother and father; however, he decided to stay with the themes she raised regarding her father. This was because he was the central figure in her story, and the question of how best to be with her father was most immediate to her. Jim followed Lee's lead in the way that she wanted to tell her story, while being mindful of helping her consider how those relationships impacted her caring for her father.

Upon reflection, Ed – the one who seems not to have been a 'recipient' of any direct spiritual care – seems almost forgotten in this case. We considered this and concluded that we might have spoken to him in order to connect with him and to assess what he needed spiritually. Yet, due to his limited involvement with his father while at the Veterans Centre, there was little opportunity to engage Ed or offer him spiritual care. However, after the anointing, Ed did express gratitude to Jim for the sacrament and for his part in it. We let Ed know that spiritual support was available for him if he wanted it; however, he did not seek it.

Working collaboratively as chaplains, we supported one another in providing care to Andrew and Lee, and to Andrew's healthcare team. The benefits of the interventions we employed in addressing Andrew's and Lee's spiritual needs were affirmed by Lee's statement:

> I was deeply moved and honoured after reading the case study that you have written regarding the spiritual care that was provided to my father, myself and to my family. I will be comforted always in the way that my father's legacy is being remembered. From this experience I learned that I can pass the spiritual care that I received along to others in my life, and to encourage them to seek it when needed. I believe spiritual care is just as important as medical care.

In addition, we both collaborated closely with the healthcare team, who relied on our insights and support around Andrew's care and Lee's concerns. The comprehensive level of spiritual care we provided allowed for an outcome that impacted positively on the overall care Andrew received from his healthcare team. We engaged Lee in ways that supported her to find new possibilities to move forward in her life in more self-accepting ways.

References

Bell, V. and Troxel, D. (2001) 'Spirituality and the person with dementia: A view from the field.' *Alzheimer's Care Quarterly 2*, 2, 31–45.

Dein, S. and Stygall, J. (1997) 'Does being religious help or hinder coping with chronic illness? A critical literature review.' *Palliative Medicine 11*, 4, 291–298.

Hermann, C. (2001) 'Spiritual needs of dying patients: A qualitative study.' *Oncology Nursing Forum 28*, 1, 67–72.

Kneller, G.F. (1971) *Introduction to the Philosophy of Education*. New York, NY: John Wiley and Sons.

McClain, C.S., Rosenfeld, B. and Breitbart, W. (2003) 'Effect of spiritual well-being on end-of-life despair in terminally-ill cancer patients.' *Lancet 361*, 9369, 1603–1607.

Orchard, H. and Clark, D. (2001) 'Tending the soul as well as the body: Spiritual care in nursing and residential homes.' *International Journal of Palliative Nursing 7*, 11, 541–546.

Russell, S. and Carey, M. (2004) *Narrative Therapy: Responding to Your Questions*. Adelaide, Australia: Dulwich Centre Publications.

Shamy, E. (2003) *A Guide to the Spiritual Dimension of Care for People with Alzheimer's Disease and Related Dementia*. London: Jessica Kingsley Publications.

Smith, S.D.M. (2005) 'Dementia palliative care needs assessment: A focus on spiritual care.' *Scottish Journal of Healthcare Chaplaincy 8*, 1, 13–19.

White, M. (2007) *Maps of Narrative Practice*. New York, NY: W.W. Norton.

Wilson, S.A. and Daley, B.J. (1999) 'Family perspectives on dying in long-term care settings.' *Journal of Gerontological Nursing 25*, 11, 19–25.

WHO (2002) *National Cancer Control Programmes: Policies and Managerial Guidelines* (2nd edn). Geneva: World Health Organization.

Chapter 12

'What can you do for me?'

– David, a mid-sixties Jewish man with stage IV pancreatic cancer

Nina Redl

Introduction

The following case unfolded several years ago during my time as chaplain in a hospital in East Jerusalem. The medical system in Israel is full of extremes. Despite large and world-renowned medical centres, a large part of the lower-income population, and all those without sufficient access to health insurance, rely on small neighbourhood clinics. These clinics are often barely more than shacks with a few mattresses and basic field medical equipment. The country's complicated politics make it either undesirable or impossible for non-Jewish, poor or illegal people to be admitted to the bigger medical facilities found in cities such as Jerusalem, Tel Aviv and Haifa.

I am a conservative rabbi and board certified chaplain, born and raised in Germany. After finishing my academic studies in the US, I took a break and spent time in Israel, where I had taken a part-time teaching position and served as a volunteer chaplain. I had gone into chaplaincy from a background of working in underserved, underdeveloped settings. Having a background in nursing and in chaplaincy, I decided to volunteer as a chaplain (in Hebrew, *tomekhet ruchanit*, the supporter of the soul/spirit). I had no fixed work hours, full freedom to engage pastorally in whatever way I saw fit, with the only responsibility to be available to any patient, staff member, family member and volunteer, as needed.

At the time I worked on this case, the pastoral care done in hospitals rested in the hands of community clergy and lay volunteers. On the Christian side, some hospitals were run by monastic orders, and their patients received religious support from staff and volunteers. Additionally, Christian clergy would visit their congregants in other hospitals. On the Jewish side, Jewish clergy and laypeople embraced the *halakhic* (Jewish law) commandment of visiting the sick (*bikkur cholim*) in a formalized and institutionalized way. Interfaith chaplaincy was nascent with initiatives by NAJC Israel and private initiatives such as Kashuvot. As a profession, chaplaincy was mostly unknown or unrecognised by the Israeli government and paid jobs were only available as hired a kind of 'pastoral therapist'.

The hospital I worked at was the middle ground. A small, old building with a few trained nurses, doctors and volunteers, its mission was, and is, towards chronic and end-of-life care; hence, medical treatment for acute conditions was very limited. The patient population encompassed a few dozen patients, primarily geriatric, oncology, HIV and other chronic and terminal illnesses. Patients were Christian, Christian-Arab, Jewish and Muslim, as were the staff. It was a good place to be when dying, and a place for healing, but most often not for cure. Upon meeting with the hospital's director, it was clear to me that this was a place where I wanted to work.

This is where I met David, a Jewish man in his mid-sixties, brought up Orthodox in the old city of Jerusalem. David was the oldest of three children. He grew up speaking Hebrew, Yiddish and Arabic fluently. His friends were Jewish, Christian and Muslim children alike, as is not uncommon in the old city. Even though there is the division of the quarters, while he grew up he experienced little division or separation between the people who lived there. Despite the political tensions and the constant struggles, David had a rather typical upbringing. Like many children that consider the old city their world, he barely ever left the old city walls.

Yet David's early adult years were interrupted by one of the not infrequent street bombings. This time his mother was killed, and it was David, as the oldest son, who had to identify her and deliver the news to his family. Shortly afterwards, his father committed suicide. From then on, 16-year-old David became the head of the family, raising his younger siblings and taking over his father's business as a shoemaker. When the business no longer brought in enough money, he was forced to close it. For a few years, he took any available job to keep himself and his siblings' heads above water. Eventually, his siblings grew up and left home. David, however, found himself unable to move on and realize his dreams. He married but never felt close to his wife. Eventually, they divorced. Finally, he became a low-paid bank clerk and occasional housekeeper, working inside a sterile and industrial environment that could not be more opposite of that to which he was accustomed.

When I met him, David had recently been diagnosed with stage IV pancreatic cancer. He had been told that there was no curative treatment for him. Since he had had to face more physical pain than he could function with while living by himself, he had decided to come to the hospice part of our hospital, primarily for palliative and end-of-life care.

David died during my first few months working in the hospice; hence, gaining his permission to tell and publish his story was impossible. Never having met his family, and not being able to reach them even through his old hospital records, I could gain permission only from the hospital director to tell David's story under the condition that I use a pseudonym, generalize his story and leave out any details that could identify him to the reader.

Case study

The first time I saw David, I barely recognized him as a patient. My initial thought was that this middle-aged man had to be a family member who had finished a visit. There was an energy about him, a strength that was palpable, despite his slow walk. The patients around me seemed to know him quite well, and he stopped briefly to joke with some of them in Arabic. The only detail about his appearance that I could not place was that he seemed to suck on two lollipops. Given the excessive drug, tobacco and candy culture of the neighbourhood, I didn't think about it twice, even though it made me silently chuckle to see a grown man with what I deemed to be children's sweets.

Seeing him standing there, grinning through his lollipops, made me think that, despite his obvious age, he had not lost a childlike joy. Unfortunately, he was neither a relative nor visitor, but a patient suffering from rapidly growing, end-stage pancreatic cancer. The lollipops were actually narcotics. He seemed to be coming and going as he liked, not paying attention to any hospital regulations and structures other than medication times. There was a sense of fierce independence about him. I attempted several times to speak to him when I saw him passing, but to no avail. The most I would get was a searching look or a sneer before he turned around. This reaction roused my sense of curiosity. A couple of days later, I stopped him in the hallway.

Chaplain: Hi, David, I am Nina.

David: (*Looking at me quizzically*) And who would you be? What can you do for me?

Chaplain: I am the *tomekhet ruchanit* here, and I thought you might want someone to talk to.

David: Spiritual…you mean like religion?

Chaplain: Yes, that is one part of what I do: I have time to listen, and if you would like, we can pray together.

David: Ahh, nonsense, religion is bad. Don't you see what it has done to this country – to all of us?

He spat on the floor, hit the wall with his fist and left without even looking at me. His blunt way of turning down my attempt to connect with him, and his strong reaction to even the mention of religion, startled me. I retreated to watching him again. I figured I needed to get a picture of him before I could attempt again to connect with him.

David clearly had an angry side to him. I witnessed several verbal fights he had with one of the doctors which demonstrated his wish to control his own medication and not follow their advice. His outbursts came suddenly, were borderline violent, but then resolved as if they had never happened.

Despite his tension with staff, David seemed to enjoy following the medical team around. At times he appeared to be the constant shadow of the nurses and doctors. Regularly, during early-morning rounds, he could be found leaning in the doorway in the nursing office, listening with concentration, positioning himself in a way that, if it hadn't been for his non-medical clothing, one could have easily mistaken him for a member of the medical team. When being denied this role, he would burst out in anger, curse and respond with very obvious gestures. When I asked my team why he was coming and going as he liked, I got the answer, 'Well, that's just him. There's nothing we can do. He knows no boundaries, and you better not come between him and what he wants – or he will rip your head off!' Over time, he had grown to be both feared and pitied by the staff.

Late one evening, when I passed by his room, I heard someone moaning. Not knowing whether it came from him, I entered only to find the curtain around David's bed drawn shut. When I carefully peeked inside, I got a furious look that communicated very clearly, 'Get out and leave me alone!' I learned from the medical team that, as he often did, he had overmedicated during the day and could not be given any more pain medication, except intravenously, which he adamantly refused.

In over a month, David had had no visitors. His trips outside the hospital had gotten shorter and shorter, and at night the moaning went on longer and longer. So far, all my attempts to connect to him had resulted in him sneering at me or simply ignoring me. Knowing I would not be able to connect with him during the day, I started a different strategy. Due to pain and overmedication, David's nights were still the most complicated time of his day. I supposed the quiet time brought up memories and thoughts of what lay ahead of him. I started staying longer into the evenings in the hospital, sitting just outside his room, close to the little coffee and tea station where patients and families could prepare themselves something to drink. I found that at least once every evening he would come and get a strong cup of black tea. In the beginning, I was afraid he would turn around and leave the moment he saw me, but I hoped at the same time that being there, without being intrusive, allowing for a few moments of being together in the same place, without actively doing anything, might give me a way of being around David that he would find acceptable. After a few days of my being there, David actually began to take more time to make his tea, even accepting the sugar and spoon I had prepared for him on the little table so that, despite his shaking hands, he could go through his tea ritual without interruption. We never said a word, nor did we look at each other. It was as if evening by evening the language we used was the actions that went into preparing a cup of tea. Once his tea was brewed and mixed, he immediately disappeared again into his room, his moaning often slowly subsiding.

After one long weekend that I had spent away from the hospital, the first message I got from one of my nurses was, 'David is waiting for you; you must come to the balcony right away'. It came to me as a complete surprise, but I hoped at the same time that maybe the few quiet moments we had shared in each other's presence may have shifted how he related to me – a thought that I barely dared to entertain. Walking out there, I sat next to him, and for a good while neither of us spoke a word. For the first time during the daytime, I could not feel the aura of challenge or anger around him. It was as if we continued our silent night-time conversations, but this time in broad daylight – and without tea.

David: I do not like to talk to people.

Chaplain: I could tell.

David: And I still don't like to.

Chaplain: You don't have to. (*silence*) But you shout pretty well for someone who does not like to say anything…and you talk in other ways than just with words.

He looked at me startled. I almost feared I would now be the target for his next outburst.

David: Well said, *habibti* [my friend]. (*He turned around and smiled.*) Come!

He stood up and went to the edge of the balcony. He pointed towards the old city.

David: This is where I am from…over there. Have you been to the old city yet?

Chaplain: Yes, I have, many times.

David: Ahh, but you don't know it…not the way I do.

Chaplain: Then why don't you tell me about it?

I was incredibly relieved; he had given me an opening into his world. He had reached out, even if it was only to challenge and test me, and I seemed to have passed his initial test. For the next hour, David talked and started to share his story with me – parts in Hebrew, parts in Arabic, a few English words in between. Seeing him standing there at the edge of the balcony, looking towards his place of birth in the old city, he seemed to grow and transform into a healthier, younger and stronger version of himself. People born and raised in the old city of Jerusalem, no matter what quarter, are not just Jerusalemites. They proudly consider themselves the real inhabitants of the city, the heart of this ancient place. Listening to David, seeing his pride and love for his city and country embodied in his every word, his story and parts of the history of Jerusalem came alive.

Over the next few weeks, I spent more time with David, sometimes talking, sometimes just sitting with him. Sometimes we traded languages: I taught him some English, he taught me some Arabic. After our first long conversation, he had let me know that he would not mind my company, even if he was not ready to talk. Just like in our early encounters at night, the silence was filled. When he got up and walked away, I often heard a whispered '*Shukran*' (Thank you).

I started to realize that when David spoke about events that hurt him, his voice rose – his anger and feelings of abandonment found a very loud way out. These expressions were often accompanied by gestures and, in the beginning, by hitting objects in his way. I attributed that to his having had to hold his anger, fear and frustrations inside for decades. When talking to me about those hard times of his life, the words abandonment and loneliness were prevalent. His life experience had been one of being alone – feeling abandoned by his parents, siblings, wife, God, country and now finally by his body, which was slowly succumbing to cancer. He had experienced a lifetime of hurt to which he reacted with anger. Over time, he shared how what he was left with was nothing *but* anger – anger at a world where seemingly there was no place for his dreams; anger at a country so shaken by instability and conflicting politics that his fate went unnoticed and was at times almost belittled.

David was surprisingly well versed in talking about his feelings, mostly in Arabic. Under the crust of hurt, fuming anger and artificial indifference, I found self-awareness and a refined way of looking at the world and himself, as well as an overall wisdom. This became particularly clear when he talked about his family of origin and the hurt, grief and loss around his parents. With a stoking voice, hoarse and often very slow, he would tell me of that hurt, grief and loss, particularly as it related to his father's suicide, which had caused him to lose trust in all emotional relationships. As a young adult, he had decided not to trust or feel anymore – to live his life without feelings so that he would not hurt anymore. He shared how he had become intensely aware that trying to carry out this decision had not only caused him more hurt, it had also made it, over the years, increasingly impossible to connect with others.

At first, the staff kept their distance from us, only briefly interrupting at medication times; however, as the days went by, the male staff members especially started approaching carefully. Not only had the atmosphere around David started to become more gentle (in step with him growing weaker through the progression of his illness), staff also began seeing him more as a person than an interruption and a burden. At times, while sitting on the balcony, they would join us for a cup of tea or coffee, a cigarette or a water pipe. Knowing the confidence and trust David put in me by telling me many details of his story, I supported this process by advocating for him with the staff. With his permission, I shared some facts about the development of David's life as they pertained to his reactions and his view of his illness, treatment and outlook towards the end of his life. Slowly he grew closer to some staff members as I helped him share some of his story in a safe space with them.

What stood out to me was that, while still forcefully requesting a high amount of pain medication at every possible opportunity, during our times together David could go for hours without a lollipop or a pain pill. It seemed that, as much as he needed the opioids for his growing physical pain, he also used them to medicate his feelings of fear, anger and sadness. He numbed his emotional and spiritual pain at times when he was not willing to deal with it.

Over the last few weeks of his life, David's pain was out of control, and almost nothing short of semi-sedation could bring him relief; however, during our time together he would demand not to be under too much pain medication so that he could converse and think straight. He shared that when talking about what really mattered to him, his physical pain would seem to ease. This helped me and the medical team realize that a considerable amount of his physical pain was existential: his pain did not only result from the cancer, but was much more from his sense of abandonment by his family and God, his loneliness and lack of purpose. When this was addressed, during our meetings he was able to let go of some of the pain that was inside his soul and thus experience ease of physical symptoms.

In his last days, a staff member would always be with him, and during his final hours, he was surrounded by the staff and volunteers to whom he had grown closer. He was minimally sedated upon his own wish; the mere presence of people who now genuinely cared for him was enough to ease his pain of dying and loneliness.

Discussion

Assessment and interventions

David had been traumatized by the violent death of his parents and by the sudden, radical onset of adulthood, and never had time to deal with, or find healing from, the trauma. The nurturing environment that teaches a young person how to become an adult had been taken away from him; instead, he was the one who had to nurture and raise his siblings. In his mind, society had failed him, and his new role isolated him from all he had known before. The bond to his siblings became all he had left, but it was complicated through his new role. When they grew up, David found himself unable to pick up his own life. Being left behind again, the only role he had known, that of a caretaker, disintegrated. Once again, he felt abandoned. Because of being unable to bear being alone, he became a husband and found himself in a marriage that he was not ready for, because he had never learned to be interdependent.

Upon the breakdown of this marriage, David withdrew into isolation. He had embraced fierce independence all his life, and paid the price in loneliness and retreat into feelings of hurt and anger. His illness became just another stroke against him, another proof that his life was not fair, yet another obstacle to tackle by himself – except that this time, he knew the cancer would win. The risk of being left or hurt meant that voluntary, lonely independence was better than taking the risk of ever getting close to someone again. It was how he had constructed his social reality. Still, it was almost impossible not to notice how much he longed not to be alone.

FROM A SILENT SAFE SPACE TO A LIFE REVIEW

From the first time we met, David's presence seemed to be filled with anger, hurt and frustration that went deep and beyond words. It was clear to me that it was not with words that the first connection needed to be formed. It was through the simple intentional coexistence of two presences in one space, what Miller and Cutshall (2001) call a 'healing presence', 'being consciously and compassionately in the present moment with another or with others, believing in and affirming their potential for wholeness, wherever they are in life' (p.12). And it was exactly that coexistence of another presence that David had denied, consciously and unconsciously, to everyone around him. Being amongst people, but being socially isolated and not part of a team, group or family, had been his life story (Weiss 1973, 1987). Wondering where in his life this amount of anger and hurt came from, I hoped that giving David a chance to tell his story and to do a life review would be a successful intervention. Telling his story became not just a life review, but an exploration into his emotional and spiritual history as he relived the emotions of his past. The moments of physical and emotional death and despair in his life were plenty; chances to grieve and experience moments of healthy connection were few. Helping him step out of this loneliness and see that a caring connection could be possible, without losing himself or feeling abandoned again, was one of my first goals for the pastoral relationship.

His prevalent anger, grief and despair were the first emotions I addressed. Despair and anger were interconnected triggers in his life. Being forced to grow up at a very early stage in his life, he survived by being fiercely independent, yet subconsciously he longed for companionship. This internal dynamic made the hospital and its staff both a desirable anchor and another unsafe space for him. Hence, my intention in being with David was to try to create an emotionally safe space that would allow for all of his emotions to be present without direct or implicit punishment; a place to let out his feelings of loneliness without being alone; a place where he could experience some continuity of spiritual and emotional care. Seeing that this was not possible by simply inviting him with words, I demonstrated it by being present and insistent, silently showing that I would not be easily scared off by his behaviour. My impression was that his aggressive outbursts expressed not just anger, but a certain kind of testing: Who would be able to stand up to him? Who would be caring and worthy enough to be with him in his worst moments? At times, I had the impression that he intentionally exaggerated his outbursts just to see how people would react. After a lifetime of loss and of being abandoned physically, spiritually and emotionally, he would not easily be convinced that people would remain caring, especially when – in his eyes – it was their professional responsibility to care. Pushing them away meant not having to let them in; repeatedly confirming to himself that no one could pass his test, he was sustained in the only security he hung onto: that he would remain abandoned. Still, deep down it seemed that he desperately wanted someone to pass his test. In hiding, there was the need to be found.

Our 'tea ritual' helped him ease into a safe space. Night-time was David's most vulnerable time, and I knew I was taking a risk trying to connect with him at this particular time of day, given that he could very well have shut down even more. My presence in the tea area could have robbed him of the safe space of his night-time wanderings, and I hoped I would be sensitive to whether that was the case. The need for safety and connection is highest when at times of vulnerability, and I hoped that David's need for connection would outweigh my intrusion. Furthermore, I hoped that, when at night his defensive mechanism decreased due to weakness and pain, a space could open up that would normally have been blocked. Since in the beginning of our tea encounters there were no words, the sacredness of the silence and the safety of it could be allowed. I hoped my presence would communicate a simple message: 'I am here. I will not be scared off, either by pain or by anger. I will not force you to talk or engage, but I can wait until you are ready to reach out.' Knowing how precious these few moments were, that a silent connection and initial trust was being established, I left the initiative of how and whether he wanted to proceed in David's hands, and just a few days later, he did reach out, actively and with words. The safe space that started with silence could then be trusted to endure words.

After our first conversation on the balcony, I could feel his need to talk and, at the same time, his fear of letting someone into his story. I decided to check in with him whenever we ran into each other, keeping my greetings casual but offering him the possibility to talk. When he did talk, I initially only asked factual questions so as to show my real curiosity about him, but without pushing him to reflect, feeling that he first needed to get his story out in his own way. It was when he started making eye contact, searching out my company and thanking me, that I knew that my careful approach in letting him take the lead was working. It was a great relief, since often, during our conversations, I had felt tempted to challenge and go deeper, but I decided not to go there before he was ready to share what he needed to share. It was a risk I took, knowing that maybe he would close up again after he had spoken, but the risk of alienating him by pushing too early seemed greater. I decided that, if all he needed was to tell his story his way, this would already be a success given that he had never done that before with someone else. Often, I had to differentiate between my own need to go deeper with him and his initial need of just telling what he decided to tell, so I adjusted my pace to his process.

BEING THE LESSER SIDE OF TRAGIC

David lived in a country that is filled with tragedy on an everyday basis; a country whose people are worn out by war and conflict. He lived in a sociopolitical situation where similar things happen to so many people that his story was not even recognized as tragic. There is hardly anyone who has not lost a loved one or a family member in one of the wars, fights and riots of the past 70 years. There is a good part of the population that still has vivid memories of the *Shoa* (Holocaust). There are many people who are their family's sole survivor, be that of the Second World War or of one of the many other wars and uproars. If one were inclined to compare tragedies, David's story would fade into the background and, as he was frequently told by friends and neighbours, he was not as badly off as others – he at least still had a house and a few family members left and, before his cancer, had been physically healthy.

Having a healthy life with a 'normal' course is still something that is rather new in Israel, unless one belongs to the financially well-off immigrant population from Western Europe or the US. Being special often means being special in a tragic way. The way David longed to be special was to be normal (i.e. trauma-free, with a predictable and regulated way of life). Lacking the 'normality' he desired, but not being sufficiently traumatized to be counted as 'special', David received no recognition or support; by the standards of his traumatized society, he was comparatively normal, but it was not 'normal' in the way he needed to be. He belonged neither to the 'larger-than-life crisis group' nor to the 'normal group'; hence, he never had a chance to find equilibrium in his life, either for his reactions or for his emotions and actions. Experiencing extreme dependence and independence were normal for him; having interdependence, or a relationship that was mutual on all existential levels, was something he had never experienced. Both his dependence and his independence put him in a space of being alone and isolated. His terminal cancer diagnosis eventually just confirmed what he had experienced all his life: tragedy, isolation and hopelessness, with the only difference being that now, all of a sudden, his body had 'betrayed' him and he could not fight through it. This triggered anger and fear. His reaction was to fight and push the boundaries he thought he was able to control: refusing the role of being a 'patient'; reaching for relationships on an equal level with the staff that were simply impossible by hospital standards; pushing everyone away who could be a resource to him. The hospital structure offered him a space for healing, but since no cure could be offered, he was not able to accept that he could experience healing in a structured environment. Recognizing this lifelong dynamic, and how it played out during his hospitalization at the end of his life, showed me the importance of helping him with his life review – making sure that what he went through was recognized as traumatic and deserving of attention and healing. Spiritual care in this situation meant treating him as not only special but unique in a healthy way.

SPIRITUALITY AND RELIGION

The English word 'spirit' is derived from the Latin *spiritus*. Its primary translation is breath, and it is used in ancient and medieval medical writings to describe the physical activity of breathing (e.g. *spiritus lenis* = light/easy breathing, *spiritus asper* = hard/laboured breathing) (Lewis and Short 2002). However, *spiritus* has a secondary translation as 'life force', 'spirit' and 'energy', and it is this translation that has found primary place in theological literature. I define spirituality broadly, based on its primary translation as 'breath'. For me spirituality is not just religious, nor is it bound to a belief in a higher power. Rather, it entails everything that makes us breathe and breathe freely, everything that defines us and identifies us. Hence, I believe everyone has a form of spirituality, whether it be related to something sacred or something profane; even the profane becomes 'sacred' if it makes us feel alive and gives us the power to go through challenging situations.

In keeping with this definition, giving David a chance to connect, experience emotional safety and healthy relationships, to live in a safe space both physically and emotionally for the end of his life, as well as helping and allowing him to relive his life story and wrestle with it, gave him a chance for partial healing in a situation where neither a physical cure nor full emotional and spiritual healing were possible; hence, this was a long-term (almost 4 months) spiritual intervention.

For the religious aspect, the following needs to be understood: For almost anyone growing up in the Middle East, religion is a part of their lives. Most people have a much stronger background in Judaism, Islam and Christianity than in the western world, simply by living in a country that has these three religions in their strongest forms as part of its normal landscape. Even people who describe themselves as secular do so with a large cultural background in any or all of these religions. Their knowledge of, and acculturation in, any of the religions surpasses that of a western secular person. Religion is everywhere: on the street, in the politics, in the history and in pretty much every publicly discussed topic. It is impossible to escape it. Personal religiosity or spirituality still is chosen, even though many more people adopt it simply by living in this environment. David had experienced this environment from his birth. He had struggled with religious politics and political religious fundamentalism, and with the manipulation that tears his home country apart every day. Despite not practising religion, it remained a part of his everyday life and, because of this, when the religious views of his childhood did not withstand a crisis, it became another element contributing to his loneliness.

Given how rejected he experienced himself to be by the religious communities, it is understandable that he rejected them – and their God. He never rejoined a religious community. In the light of his other, deeply existential problems, I did not focus on religion once he told me that it did not matter to him. Only towards the end of his days did he trust me enough to bring up God and allow me to bring in a Torah reading. Given the late stage of his illness, I did not push for more active religious chaplaincy work with him but instead let him chose how much he wanted to engage in, which was not a lot due to his physical and mental weakness. Still there was a sacredness and almost divine presence whenever he was in community with hospital staff at his bedside – my staff also shared in the wonder. God was present, and it was hard to doubt that David did not feel it – some things are beyond words. In a way, and even if it cannot be proven, I dare say that through some of his healing process, not just other people but *God* re-entered his life. Nevertheless, I am left wondering if I had brought up the topic of God earlier, and had more intentionally explored it with him, whether a more explicit reconciliation with his religion and God could have been reached, especially given that, to my own personal regret, a reconciliation with his family remained out of the question.

Outcomes

Even before being able to tell his story, the most important outcome of our connection was that David was able to make a connection beyond his anger. I experienced David's ability to allow himself to enter this safe space as an initial success on which we could build. It was a first sign that, despite all the hurt, he had not yet lost the ability to trust. Building a basis of trust, first without words, and then testing this trust by telling his story and finding the trust reaffirmed, was important to David's regaining of trust: first a trust in himself; then a trust in others.

He was able to experience that not only was his story heard, but also that he was accepted as a whole person, with his strengths *and* weaknesses. It was not surprising to me that David started with telling me about his home. He started his story from a place of strength and safety: the memories of his home and his early childhood. Only after that did he allow himself to share more hurtful memories. By demonstrating his strength with pride, he could 'control' my impression of him as a strong, proud and determined man, rather than as someone who was lonely, in pain, weak and dying of cancer. Showing me who he was and how he preferred to think of himself, he could then allow his vulnerability and 'dark sides' to enter the picture. His storytelling morphed into a much deeper process that had a revealing and healing character, the story of how his life seemed nothing but a painful failure to him. It was a story that, in his experience, no one ever wanted to hear – not even David himself. He had blocked a lot of it even from himself. But importantly, he was able to look at his life without being completely worn down by resignation and despair. He was able to rebuild some self-worth that was more than just bitter pride.

The life review we did helped him struggle with the inevitability of his imminent death, given that being recognized in his sadness, grief and trauma took away some of his edge to fight everything and everyone just to get attention. Sharing some of his story with staff, through me and by himself, helped him connect and experience a few caring connections, even if they were only short term. David was cared for because of, and despite, his experiences.

This narrative journey helped him be with himself, in his past and in his present and, finally, it allowed others back into his presence. Over the last few weeks of his life he formed companionships with some staff members. Obviously, the hospital was never able to replace the home he had lost, but it did become a place where he could feel safe and at times at home, surrounded by people whom he could trust, talk to and, once he was no longer mobile, allow to take care of him. When he died, David was surrounded by staff who took turns being with him until his last moment. His loneliness had been alleviated to a substantial degree, and his worst fear of dying as lonely as he had lived was not realized.

Conclusion

One of the most striking elements in the pastoral care relationship with David was how it seemed to influence his pain levels. Almost every pain comes with suffering, and I differentiate here between pain as the physical experience and suffering as the emotional and spiritual response to physical pain and other life-disrupting circumstances. Being an end-stage pancreatic cancer patient, it was to be expected that David would experience an increasing amount of pain. From the beginning, David advocated strongly for a high dose of pain medication, to which no one objected. In his case, it was hard to tell what caused him more suffering, the pain from his cancer or the feelings connected to his life story and current circumstances.

When David told me that he had never had a pain-free life (meaning free of physical pain), looking at it from an existential point of view, I was not surprised. He had suffered many losses and 'died several deaths' long before he was diagnosed with a terminal illness. All these losses and all his suffering had found physical outlets throughout his life, but it was not until he was diagnosed with terminal cancer that the compounded grief and suffering, accumulated throughout his life, started hitting him in the most physical ways. His existential pain had turned physical and was joined by the cancer pain. Yet, while talking to me about topics that were clearly emotionally loaded and hurtful, not only did he forget to ask for pain medication (as he would otherwise do on an hourly basis), he would often not take any medication at all during and after our sessions. The topics we talked about were clearly emotionally very difficult, and I could watch his physical reaction to them. When speaking about some of his deepest feelings and fears, his body would react – his hands would clench and his body would shake; often he would hug himself and rock backwards and forwards; his stomach pain would come back – but he would not ask for medication, claiming that his physical pain was 'bearable and important'. It was important pain for him to go through in order to start healing. The suffering of his soul was reflected in physical pain, but for the first time not in a destructive way – in a healing way. A large part of the pain he was feeling was not only physical, cancer-related pain, but the physical pain caused by his emotions while remembering and processing. Alleviating his existential pain, and helping him to look at his life, suffering and pain in a safe and healing environment, helped him deal with the existential side of his pain.

References

Lewis, C.T. and Short, C. (2002) *A Latin Dictionary: Based on Andrews's Edition of Freund's Latin Dictionary*. (Original work published 1879.) Available at www. perseus.tufts.edu/hopper/text?doc=Perseus:text:1999.04.0059, accessed on 4 July 2014.

Miller, J.E. and Cutshall, S.C. (2001) *The Art of Being a Healing Presence*. Fort Wayne, IN: Willow Green Publishing.

Weiss, R.S. (1973) *Loneliness: The Experience of Emotional and Social Isolation*. Cambridge, MA: MIT Press.

Weiss, R.S. (1987) 'Reflections on the present state of loneliness research.' In M. Hojat and R. Crandall (eds) *Loneliness: Theory, Research and Applications* (pp. 1–16). Thousand Oaks, CA: SAGE.

Chapter 13

'Tell her that it's OK to release her spirit'

– Maria, a Native American woman, grieving the loss of her dying mother

Richard C. Weyls

Introduction

Esmeralda was an 85-year-old Native American ('First Nations') woman who was admitted to the hospital after an incident of acute respiratory failure and subsequent pulse-less, electrical-activity cardiac arrest. The patient also had a history of severe chronic obstructive pulmonary disease, carbon dioxide retention (hypercapnia) and aortic stenosis. She had struggled with chronic illness for many years but had been doing quite well at home during the previous year. The patient's quality of life had been acceptable to her, and she had enjoyed spending time with her large extended family. Esmeralda was a revered elder in her family and Native American clan. She shared her 'Native ways' with the younger generations through storytelling, singing and teaching. Because of her relatively good health, Esmeralda had not seen her primary care physician during the previous year.

While shopping with her daughter, Esmeralda had become quite fatigued and asked to return home to rest. She became increasingly lethargic and began to experience respiratory distress. Her family members called for emergency medical assistance. As they were waiting for help to arrive, the patient stopped breathing. Cardiopulmonary resuscitation (CPR) was not administered by family members, but her daughter attempted mouth-to-mouth resuscitation. Five minutes later, the emergency medical technicians arrived, performed full CPR, regained a pulse and intubated the patient. Esmeralda arrived at the emergency department in cardiac arrest. She was revived with CPR and electrocardioversion. She was resuscitated three times in the emergency department before becoming stable enough to transfer to the cardiac intensive care unit (ICU).

Many of Esmeralda's family members were present during the numerous resuscitative efforts. Though shocked and fearful, they were supportive of the plan of care. The admitting physician wrote that 'the patient's overall condition is very complex and prognosis is grim'. As the day progressed, Esmeralda showed signs of clinical deterioration and possible anoxic central nervous system injury. The intensive care physician informed the family that it was very unlikely that Esmeralda would survive and return to her former functional status. The family members accepted that she was declining, and they were concerned that current medical efforts might be prolonging the dying process. Esmeralda's loved ones did not wish for her to undergo CPR and electrocardioversion again. They were afraid that Esmeralda might be suffering. After consulting extensively with one another and the attending physician, the family requested that Esmeralda's code status be changed to 'do not resuscitate' to allow for a natural death. This all transpired within the first 12 hours of Esmeralda's hospitalization. No spiritual care provider or chaplain had been involved in Esmeralda's care to this point.

Surprisingly, Esmeralda survived the night in the ICU. The family members, represented by Esmeralda's daughter, Maria, expressed their desire to withdraw life-sustaining treatment in order to allow for a natural death. They contacted the unit chaplain to request faith-specific, culturally unique rituals for the dying. Maria explained that her mother was 'culturally Native and religiously Catholic'. They requested sacramental ministry from a Roman Catholic priest and special death rituals from a Native Holy Man. My primary relationship was with Maria, a proud, grieving, middle-aged woman with graying hair, and her son, Melchior. Their large, multigenerational family also played a significant role.

I am a middle-aged Caucasian male, of mostly European descent, who was ordained as a Roman Catholic priest in 1993. One of my distant relatives was a member of a First Nations people in Ontario, Canada (probably Algonquin), but I do not identify with my Native roots. I am a citizen of the United States and have awareness of my Irish, Welsh and Slovak heritage. I completed one unit of clinical pastoral education (CPE) as a seminarian and served as a sacramental minister for several acute care hospitals in the Midwest while working as a parish priest. I provided leadership in parish ministry for 15 years until resigning from the priesthood in 2008 due to personal, professional and theological reasons. I completed a residency in hospital chaplaincy in 2010 and became a board certified chaplain with the Association of Professional Chaplains in 2011. As part of my chaplaincy training, I have completed a total of six units of CPE through the Association of Clinical Pastoral Education. I am endorsed for chaplaincy by the Episcopal Church USA (Anglican Communion), and I am in the process of having my priestly ordination recognized by the Episcopal Church.

This encounter occurred in 2009 during my CPE residency. I recorded it in a detailed verbatim format and discussed it with my CPE peers and supervisor. It touched upon much of my own personal and professional grief. It occurred when I was still actively grieving the loss of my identity and role as a Roman Catholic priest and transitioning into a new career as a professional chaplain and Episcopalian. I could not function licitly as a Catholic priest in this circumstance, and it was also not consistent with my new pastoral identity and state in life. I felt conflicted as I waited with the family over a period of hours for the Catholic priest to arrive; however, it was important to my personal and professional integrity to maintain this important boundary.

I work as a staff chaplain for Swedish Health Systems in Seattle, Washington. 'Swedish' has grown over the last 103 years to become the largest non-profit health provider in the Greater Seattle area. It is composed of five hospital campuses, two ambulatory care centers and Swedish Medical Group, a network of more than 100 primary care and specialty clinics located throughout the Greater Puget Sound area. In addition to general medical and surgical care, including robotic-assisted surgery, Swedish is known as a regional referral center, providing specialized treatment in areas such as cardiovascular care, cancer care, neuroscience, orthopedics, high-risk obstetrics, pediatric specialties, organ transplantation and clinical research.

Before submitting this case for publication, I consulted with the institutional review board of Swedish Health Systems to seek their advice about the ethical issues involved in this study. My institution defines research as 'the collection of data for the purposes of dissemination for general knowledge' (Hansberry 2013). I explained that the subject of this study died in 2009. The board representative responded that 'we generally see case studies on deceased individuals as not meeting the definition'; however, the board consented, requiring that I protect the identities of all individuals involved and comply with the Health Insurance Portability and Accountability Act of 1996. Consequently, all of the names have been changed and personal health information has been de-identified. Some of the unique details of the case have been altered or omitted in order to protect confidentiality.

Case study

It is quite common in acute care chaplaincy to encounter patients and families in a crisis situation. I did not know the patient, Esmeralda, and family before this time; I met Maria after it was determined that Esmeralda would be withdrawn from life-sustaining treatment, and the pastoral relationship formed very quickly due to an emergent need for spiritual care. Maria requested the services of a Roman Catholic priest to celebrate the Anointing of the Sick and other Catholic rituals for those in danger of death. Unfortunately, the family's parish priest was unavailable and the hospital priest-chaplain could not respond until the evening. As chaplain, I made these arrangements and visited the family several times during the period of waiting.

It was during this first encounter that I learned that the family members intended to celebrate traditional Native American death rituals, in addition to Roman Catholic 'last rites'. I quickly determined that my role, as chaplain, was to serve as host for the celebration of these different, yet complementary, end-of-life rituals. Maria informed me of their desire to enlist the help of a Native Holy Man who would do smudging (a ritual involving the burning of herbs and grasses), drumming and chanting. As a representative of the hospital, I advised Maria that they could not actively burn any herbs in the ICU for safety reasons. She was already aware of this, because the Holy Man had conducted these rituals in hospitals many times before; in fact, he had been present at the death of Maria's father about 15 years earlier. The Holy Man would adapt the rite so that the burning would take place outside the hospital at the family home. The aromatic ashes would then be used at bedside.

Rather than being a spiritual care expert or celebrant of rituals, I assumed the role of coordinator, facilitator and student. I also functioned as a representative of the hospital and served as family advocate to the nursing and medical staff. I had some familiarity with Native American customs but did not know the unique traditions of this particular Roman Catholic/Native American family system. I sensed that Maria needed to observe these rituals faithfully and teach them to others to make meaning in this time of loss.

I established a relationship of trust with Maria earlier in the day as we discussed her mother's impending death. As the day progressed, Maria became focused on the details of the desired rituals and sought my assistance to coordinate this spiritual care. I informed her that the Roman Catholic priest would arrive at the hospital in the evening.

Maria: Yes, that would be perfect. The Holy Man will be here by then too. I am still waiting for the rest of my family to arrive. They are at home removing my mother's belongings from the house. This must be done before sunset on the day she dies; otherwise, her spirit will remain captive in this plane of existence. That is why we cannot speak her name for I year after her death. If we do, her spirit will not leave us. We believe that her spirit will roam this world for I year until it is joined again to the Great Spirit.

Maria introduced me to her son, Melchior, a short, dark-haired man who appeared to be in his twenties. It seemed that his role was to support his mother in this time of loss. He proudly shared that he was named after one of the Three Kings who visited Jesus after his birth. Melchior continued to instruct me while I attempted to connect with him on a feeling level. I invited Maria to describe the rituals they intended to observe and asked how I could be of help.

Chaplain: Hello, Melchior. I imagine this is a scary and painful time for you.

Melchior: Yes. (*He begins crying.*) My grandmother is Oneida. It is a matriarchal culture. She is the head of our clan. We know that her body needs to release her spirit. She seems trapped right now. I want her to be free.

Chaplain: What a terrible loss this is for you. You must feel very helpless right now.

Melchior: I do. I am helpless to stop her physical death, but I can help her release her spirit. We need to let her go.

Chaplain: How loving and courageous you are to be willing to let her go, in spite of your own pain.

Melchior: We express our love by observing some very sacred death rituals. The Holy Man understands that we cannot burn anything in the room. He has done this many times before. He will burn the desert sage, cedar and sweet grass before he comes to the hospital.

Chaplain: I want to support you in your sacred rituals, but I'm not sure how. How can I be of help?

Maria: Our entire family will gather for the release of my mother's spirit. We will have four generations here. No one can speak her name after her death, including you, the priest or nurse. I will place these prayer bundles on her now. They are red and yellow. Yellow is the color of death. It contains a straw doll that my mother was given when she received her Indian name. It has no face. We believe that the events of her life have carved a face in the doll. We have never seen it, because it was immediately wrapped in yellow cloth and tied with string, and saved for this moment. It is placed on her during the dying process and must be cremated with her. She needs this to present herself to the Great Spirit. Please tell the nurse and others not to touch the prayer bundles. If they need to be moved for some reason, let one of the family members move them. We believe that bad things will happen to a non-Native who touches them. I don't want this to happen to anyone. You have all been so wonderful to us.

This red prayer bundle contains tobacco and prayers, written in our Native language. These must remain with the body and be cremated with her. Can you make sure this happens? After her death, it is OK to touch the bundles. Just make sure they stay with the body.

The Holy Man will do the smudging ceremony by waving the scent of the burned herbs around her body. He will also paint her face to prepare her for the final battle. We will do a lot of chanting also, especially 'The Warrior Song'.

My mother is Oneida. Her mother and father were both from the northeastern forest tribes. Her mother was Oneida. Her father was Huron. My father, her husband, was Crow. They are a plains nation. The Holy Man is Crow. He was present at my father's death 15 years ago.

We will also place a transition blanket on my mother when we do the final rituals. This very blanket has been placed on our dying ancestors for over 300 years. The Holy Man will also remove four locks of her hair before she dies. This is an Oneida tradition. One lock will be given to each female in the direct family line: me, my daughter, who is especially close to her, and my granddaughter. The last lock is for all of the women who are yet to be born in our family line.

We are of the Turtle Clan of the Oneida people. Our creation story teaches that the world sits on the back of a cosmic turtle. If you look at a turtle's shell, you can see the shape of the globe with the continents separated by water. The men of our tribe wear a tattoo of the turtle on their chests. (*Melchior shows me his tattoo.*) I have taught all of my children our Native ways. We are culturally Native and religiously Catholic. My family has been Catholic for generations. We can't begin our Native rituals until the priest does the last rites. When will he be here?

I confirmed that the priest-chaplain would arrive several hours later, in the evening. I also invited the patient's bedside nurse to join us as I summarized the aforementioned instructions. The nurse took notes and together we verified the information with Maria and Melchior. The nurse assured the family that she, personally, would accompany Esmeralda's body to the morgue to ensure that the prayer bundles remained undisturbed. She offered to pin the bundles to the patient's gown and include a note directing that the prayer bundles be cremated with the body. The nurse also crafted a sign for the door to the patient's room that read: **Family Only. Staff – Please Check with Nurse Before Entering.** She and I also informed other ICU staff of Maria's requests and reserved one of the family waiting areas for the large family that was expected throughout the day.

Maria indicated that she needed time to contact other family members and prepare for the rituals. She also wished to spend some time alone with her mother. Maria requested prayer.

Maria: Can you say some prayers with us?

Chaplain: Of course. Let's gather around your mother's bed and let her know of our love. May I invite her to pray with us?

Maria: Please do.

Chaplain: May I use her name?

Maria: Tell her that it's OK to release her spirit.

Chaplain: What name shall I use?

Maria: Use her baptismal name, Esmeralda.

Chaplain: What else would you like to pray for?

Maria: Comfort and peace.

Chaplain: Esmeralda. My name is Rich, and I am a chaplain in the hospital. I am here with your daughter, Maria, and grandson, Melchior. We are surrounding you with love right now. (*silence*)

The Catholic priest and the Native Holy Man are coming to be with you soon. We want to help you release your spirit to the Great Spirit. We will observe all of the traditional sacred rituals that you know…Catholic last rites and Native traditions.

Maria has placed two prayer bundles on you. The Holy Man will be smudging you when he gets here, and your family will be wrapping you in your family's transition blanket. There is nothing to be afraid of. Your loved ones will chant The Warrior Song for you. When Jesus comes for you, it's OK to release your spirit.

Please say these prayers with us, if you want. Even if your lips don't move, we know that you are praying with us in your heart.

Let us pray.

Great Spirit, loving Mother-God. We know you are with us as we prepare to help your beloved child release her spirit unto you. Help us to observe these sacred rituals with sincerity and devotion. Be with this loving family as they let go of their mother, grandmother and matriarch. Give them comfort, strength and peace. Ease their pain and stir up their hope. Help us all to love each other better through Christ, our Lord, Amen.

Please add your own prayers, if you'd like.

Maria: Our Father, who art in heaven...
  Hail, Mary, full of grace...
  Glory, be to the Father...
  (*Long silence and some tears.*)
  Thank you for being with us.

Chaplain: It's a privilege to be with you. Thank you for sharing your sacred rituals with me. Father should be here at about 5:30 pm. I will check in with you before then. Is there anything you might need before I go?

Maria: No, thank you. We need some time for prayer and togetherness before our work begins.

Over the next few hours I checked in with the nursing staff to see how they were coping with the large number of family members that were gathering. Esmeralda's family established a base camp in the designated lounge and did not interfere with other patients and staff. I circulated among the family members and invited them to share stories and memories of Esmeralda, while encouraging them to speak about their faith and Native American heritage. I also invited them to verbalize the multitude of emotions they were feeling: sadness, gratitude, fear, anger, confusion, love and vulnerability. Some of the more distant family members expressed guilt and regret for 'missed opportunities'. I urged small groups of family members to visit with the patient throughout the day to speak lovingly to her and say goodbye.

Eventually, I received a call from the Catholic priest-chaplain, Fr Alois, indicating that he was delayed by Seattle rush-hour traffic. He would be at least an hour late. When I communicated this to Maria, she indicated that they would proceed with the Native death rituals, since the Holy Man had arrived. She noted that the priest could join us later. Maria looked sad and emotionally exhausted. Melchior had his arm around her and was physically holding her up. I pointed out that she looked sad and tired.

Maria: I am. This is exhausting work, but it must be done.

Maria and Melchior took a place near the head of Esmeralda's bed. Esmeralda was a small, white-haired woman with a mechanical ventilator attached through an endotracheal tube. She had numerous IVs and lines connected to her frail body. Her eyes were open and her mouth was quivering. The ventilator was making her chest heave in an unnatural manner. She looked like a ventilated corpse. I felt great sadness and compassion for Esmeralda and her family. I, too, desired that the patient might 'release her spirit'.

Slowly, 17 people of various ages began drifting into the room. Most of them were in their teens and twenties. I surmised that they were grandchildren and spouses/partners. There were three small children and one infant; none looked particularly 'Native' to me. Several of the women were wearing crucifixes. The Holy Man looked like a stereotypical image of a Native American. He was tall and lean, with darker skin and strong features. His graying hair was parted in the middle with two braids on each side. He was wearing jeans, cowboy boots and a plaid shirt. He was carrying an abalone shell with burned herbs and paint. He introduced himself as Robert. I offered to help in any way. He asked me to assist him by preparing four pieces of tape. He explained that he could not locate any string or yarn. The tape would keep Esmeralda's locks of hair secure. I fastened the tape to the small cart near the bed and suggested that, as a group, we create an opportunity for the family members to say goodbye to their matriarch. He agreed.

Each family member said something to the dying woman. Many of them cried freely and sobbed. Maria collapsed on top of her mother's body. Melchior eventually eased her into a chair near the bedside.

Robert located the transition blanket from a family member. He, Maria and her daughter, Elizabeth, ceremoniously placed the blanket on the patient. Robert began the smudging ritual by waving the burned, aromatic herbs with an eagle feather toward the patient's face and body. Family members used their hands to wave the scent toward their own faces and bodies while breathing in the imaginary smoke. This was done in profound silence. As Robert began to paint Esmeralda's face, several family members began to sob and wail.

When the Holy Man finished his smudging, he invited the family to surround the bed. He stood at the foot of the bed in the middle of the group. He waited calmly until the sobbing stopped. The group became very serious. They linked arms and seemed to stand up taller than they were before. Robert began chanting in a Native language. A drum began to play with a slow, low beat. Soon the entire family began to chant. There was great energy in the room. This was The Warrior Song. At the end of the chant, there were several moments of silence. Robert began another chant, but only he and his assistant sang this one. It was much more melancholy and haunting. At the end of this song, there was a very long silence. It was clear that the ritual had ended. The silence became awkward. The family began chatting among themselves. Robert approached me and said, 'Where is the priest? She is ready to release her spirit.'

I called Fr Alois on his cell phone, only to learn that he was still 15 minutes from the hospital. I informed the family and suggested that we pray the 'Litany of the Saints' as we awaited the Father's arrival. This ancient prayer is common in several Christian denominations and is part of the Roman Catholic rite for the dying. The family members participated fully in the responses to each invocation. We included St. Esmeralda in the litany. Fr Alois arrived near the end of these prayers and joined in the responses.

Fr Alois is a native Tanzanian and a member of the Chagga people (or tribe). He told me later that he was quite comfortable with the enculturation of Native rituals with Roman Catholic rites. This was his experience as an East African, Roman Catholic tribal member. Father introduced himself and explained the shape of the rite to the family members: readings from Sacred Scripture, renewal of baptismal promises, the Apostolic Blessing, intercessory prayers, the imposition of hands, anointing with the oil of the sick, the Lord's Prayer and Prayer of Commendation. He dispensed with the Litany of the Saints since we had already prayed this. Fr Alois prompted those gathered with their responses so they could participate fully. He invited the Holy Man to stand next to him as he led the ritual. He also encouraged the Native elder and family members to lay healing hands upon Esmeralda, in silence, before the anointing with oil. A drum pounded beautifully and mournfully in the background. Many of the family members wept quietly during the rites. They all participated as they were able. After the final blessing, Melchior asked me to get the nurse and respiratory therapist to begin the withdrawal of life-sustaining treatment.

Maria and Elizabeth moved through the crowd to the head of Esmeralda's bed. Maria announced that Elizabeth would 'chant her out' to 'coax her spirit away from her body'. Elizabeth began a chant in the Native language and, eventually, Maria joined her. Soon, all of the women in the room were singing the plaintive chant. It seemed like everyone in the room was crying. At the end of the chant Maria spoke.

> *Maria:* You have been a wonderful mother. Thank you for allowing me to care for you for the past 50 years. I love you. My love releases you to the spirit world just like your love released Daddy many years ago. I release you to the Great Spirit. Jesus will be your guide.

Maria threw her head back in a loud shriek! Elizabeth joined her. Eventually, all the women joined in the blood-curdling shriek. Soon, deafening silence overtook the room. Everyone looked at the bedside monitor. The nurse turned off the alarms several times. Esmeralda had died.

The Holy Man closed Esmeralda's eyelids and began snipping off lockets of her hair. He handed them to me and asked that I secure each with tape. He whispered, 'This is an Oneida tradition.' He then gently removed the transition blanket. He folded it and gave it to Maria, who was weeping. Melchior was holding her up. Robert took the white hospital sheet and covered Esmeralda's face. He carefully repositioned the patient's hands and feet so that her entire body was fully covered. Everyone stared at the covered body in silence. Robert said, 'She has released her spirit.'

Maria stood up very tall and extracted herself from Melchior's grasp. She exuded strength and authority as the new matriarch of the clan. She made a very clear pronouncement.

Maria: Our work is done here! Thank you, Chaplain Rich, for being with us. Please tell the staff that they can touch the prayer bundles now.

Chaplain: I will make sure that they stay with your mother's body. Thank you for allowing me to be with you during this sacred time. I wish you much peace and healing. May I walk you out?

Maria: Thank you, but no. We must honor the past while we journey into the future…together. May God bless you.

The family members composed themselves, gathered their belongings and began to exit the hospital room in a quiet, unceremonious fashion. They departed the hospital in the same manner.

Discussion

Assessment

Hospital chaplains are often consulted in crisis situations. In this particular case, spiritual care was called because the family members were requesting faith-specific rituals and cultural observances. They desired the services of a Roman Catholic priest and a Native Holy Man. In evaluating and assessing the need, I asked myself the following questions:

- What is the request?

- What do they need spiritually?

- How am I able to respond?

This case was complex on many levels, but it was essentially about loss. The family members recognized that medical interventions were no longer able to yield beneficial results, and that life-sustaining treatment was prolonging the dying process. Their comments seemed to suggest that they understood the human person as an incarnate spirit. The failing human body was holding the eternal spirit 'captive', and the family members needed to celebrate rituals to help Esmeralda release her spirit to the Great Spirit. Maria, Melchior and their family were experiencing anticipatory grief, but they were also quite absorbed with 'the work' they needed to do. It became clear to me that Maria needed to engage her grief through these rituals in order to structure her reality and make meaning in this time of great loss. I determined that my role in this encounter was to serve as coordinator, facilitator and student for the celebration of some very specific death rituals. In order to analyze this more fully, I need to explain my operative theology of spiritual care, my version of spiritual assessment and some of the theory behind my work.

My theology of spiritual care is fundamentally Christian, sacramental and incarnational. I believe that through the mystery of the Incarnation (personal divinity joining itself to humanity in the person of Jesus of Nazareth) all human experiences have been touched by God from the inside. As a result, all human experiences have the capacity and potential of mediating God's grace. Divinity is intimately connected to all of creation and all things are 'in God', a version of Christian pantheism. God is supremely present in the deepest and most uniquely human experiences such as love, fear, sexuality, suffering, illness and death. I do not believe that these are merely human experiences that we ask God to visit or bless. God is already there – often more intimately than we are! The more deeply we are willing to enter into these human experiences, the more deeply we encounter God and our truest selves. These depth experiences have the capacity to reveal God's abiding presence and care for the world.

I also believe that human beings respond to this intimate, mysterious experience of God's divine presence to human life by using ritual and material things to structure their reality and make meaning. Human beings use human things (e.g. words, song, gesture, music, dance, touch) and material things (e.g. water, oil, smoke, prairie grasses, bread, wine) to enter more deeply into the mystery of the God who lives intimately in the experience itself. This is how I understand the general term 'sacrament'. I also understand relationship as sacrament.

As a chaplain I show up and offer to enter into these experiences with others. I respectfully honor their spiritual reality and invite them to go even more deeply into these experiences to encounter the God of their understanding. I walk with them as a spiritual companion and fellow pilgrim in my own search for God. I am there to learn as much as to guide. I may not have answers, but I can facilitate others' questioning as a way to enter more deeply into the mystery of God. I walk with them as a sacramental presence of God's love, compassion and healing.

This approach to spiritual care allows me to claim my own faith perspective while being open to the spiritual experiences and values of others. I work in a secular hospital that claims no particular religious affiliation; however, as an organization, we integrate spirituality into the care we offer patients and their loved ones. We affirm and embrace patients of religious faith and no faith. My theology of spiritual care allows me to serve and support people of differing spiritual and religious beliefs without threatening my own faith understanding.

In this case study, I served as a host for the unfolding of a mystery. I believed that God was truly incarnate in this unique cultural milieu. I served as facilitator for the cultural and religious rituals that the family needed to conduct in this time of loss. Maria and Melchior were quite clear and directive about what they needed in this situation. They were asking for my assistance in allowing these rituals to unfold in the cardiac ICU. I did not have the ecclesiastical authority to preside at the Roman Catholic rituals, nor the knowledge or experience to assist at the Native death customs. I tried not to assume anything. On several occasions, I asked the family members how I could be of help. Maria and Melchior were quite willing to offer guidance and direction.

I believe that my presence and behavior demonstrated my belief that 'God was there', and that this was a sacred encounter. I adapted my prayers to respect the spiritual perspective that I learned by listening to Maria describe her people's sacred death rituals. I offered a prayer to the Great Spirit and, in an attempt to honor the patient and her matriarchal culture, I addressed the prayer to 'loving Mother-God'. I also prayed, 'We know you are with us' to reflect my belief that God is intimately present in this uniquely human experience. I acknowledged their pain while inviting them to find hope in their suffering. Finally, I moved from Native imagery to more traditional language of Christian ritual to respect their Catholic faith. I experienced wonder and awe in this ministerial encounter, because I recognized it as a sacred time that revealed God's presence in a new way.

Interventions

As a spiritual care provider in the acute-care setting, I was asked to respond to a specific need. The patient was about to be withdrawn from life-sustaining treatment, and her death was imminent. The family members asked for the services of a Roman Catholic priest for faith-specific death rituals. Our hospital system retains the services of a Roman Catholic priest-chaplain for sacramental care. It was my job to make this referral. The family also needed my assistance in creating a safe space for the celebration of Native American rituals for the dying patient. This required facilitation, coordination, advocacy and a knowledge of hospital policies and culture. I interfaced with other members of the healthcare team to ensure that cultural practices were respected. I also represented the hospital regarding safety considerations (no burning or open flames in the ICU) and worked with the family to make accommodations to their rites.

Since I was responding to an emergent need, I was not able to engage the patient or family in an in-depth exploration of their spiritual beliefs. In situations such as these, I ask myself: What are they asking for? and What do they need? I did not function as a pastoral counselor or spiritual guide; rather, I showed up as a compassionate, spiritual presence that connected with the family members on an affective level, built trust and asked them to describe their ritual needs. I offered active, empathic listening, with curiosity and reverence. Maria took great pride in telling me about the cultural rituals we were about to observe. Teaching me about her heritage gave her strength and helped her cope in this time of loss. I was a humble student, companion and privileged participant as they conducted religious and cultural rituals that engaged their grief.

Another spiritual care intervention was prayer at the bedside. Maria asked that I offer a prayer to encourage the patient 'to release her spirit' and to bring 'comfort and peace' to the family. Even though the patient had suffered an anoxic brain injury, I spoke to her as if she heard and understood everything that was being said. I crafted a prayer from the deep listening I had done previously. I addressed the prayer to the Great Spirit and used maternal imagery to honor the patient, her role in the clan and the matrilineal culture. I asked for God's assistance to help Maria and her family 'observe these sacred rituals with sincerity and devotion', because I sensed this was extremely important to her. Maria seemed to need to celebrate these rituals faithfully, and teach them to her multigenerational family, before assuming her role as new matriarch. I also included traditional Catholic prayer language, with a Christological focus. I attempted to honor both the cultural milieu and the religious tradition that were operative.

I would like to suggest that additional spiritual care interventions, in this case, were my non-interference and maintenance of personal and professional boundaries. It became quite clear to me early in my encounter with this family that they needed space to celebrate rituals that would make meaning in this time of crisis and loss. Even though their experiences touched upon my own personal and professional grief, I was able to get out of the way to allow the power of the rituals to help the family express their grief, make meaning and transition to a new place in their spiritual journey. I was quite aware that this encounter was not about me and my needs. I was able to acknowledge my own feelings, honor them and use them to connect at an affective level with the people I served. In the end, I released my own struggle to God and asked for the grace to attend to my own needs at another time.

Outcomes

The spiritual care interventions in this case yielded positive outcomes for Esmeralda, her family and the hospital staff. First of all, a hospital chaplain responded to the family's request for religious and cultural death rituals. This met their perceived and requested need, which allowed the nursing and medical staff to provide expert care within their scope of practice. Showing up, and offering compassionate spiritual presence, communicated the presence of God and the care of others. Through reflective listening and empathic communication, family members were able to verbalize their many feelings and begin the initial adjustment to their significant loss. I offered prayer that honored the important cultural heritage and spiritual beliefs of the family system. This helped the family members cope with their loss and find meaning and hope.

As chaplain, I also served as a family advocate with the hospital staff and as a representative of the healthcare providers. This allowed the cultural and religious rituals to unfold with dignity and integrity while containing them appropriately in the ICU. Due to advance planning and hospitality, large numbers of family members were able to visit the patient and participate in the desired rituals without interfering with ICU activities. I tried to serve as host and facilitator for holy men of two traditions while providing support when needed. By encouraging the faithful celebration of these important rituals, Maria and family were able to acknowledge the reality of their loss, experience the pain of grief, adjust to the new environment and reinvest in a new relationship with the deceased. Other staff members offered compassionate presence, kindness and empathy to the family during this encounter; however, as chaplain, I see myself as representing God's love and healing to them. I hope that, through my pastoral identity and role, I was a sacrament of God's abiding presence and love in this time of vulnerability and pain.

From an anthropological standpoint I was intrigued by the manner in which the family members used cultural and religious rituals to engage their grief, make meaning and transition to a new place in their spiritual journey. I was reminded of the work of Arnold van Gennep (1961) and Victor Turner (1967) on rites of passage and liminality. If I were to apply these theories to this case study, I would contend that death was understood to be a rite of passage whereby Esmeralda's spirit was released to the spirit world and, ultimately, reunified with the Great Spirit. The death rituals we observed were part of the pre-liminal or *separation* stage of this rite of passage. They provided a framework for the expression of emotions and a 'letting go'. The survivors were left in the liminal or *transition* stage – a 'betwixt and between' state of ambiguity between the former stage and the *reincorporation*, or post-liminal stage, yet to come. Melchior said that 'We express our love by observing some very sacred death rituals' and, on several occasions, Maria referred to these rituals as her 'work'. Once the work was done, Maria assumed her new role as matriarch and noted that she must 'journey into the future' with her family to begin the process of reincorporation.

Conclusion

As I reflect upon and evaluate my work in this instance, I would probably do one thing differently. The praying of the Roman Catholic Litany of the Saints seemed to work well as we waited awkwardly for Fr Alois to arrive. In retrospect, I might have offered this as a way of managing my own discomfort with the pause in the rituals. The family members were chatting nervously among themselves. Today, I would probably allow them to experience and express the fullness of their anxiety rather than feeling the need to impose structured prayer upon the moment.

I was humbled and grateful to have met this family in a significant moment of pain and loss. The beautiful intersections of cultural and religious rituals were engaged in a way that allowed the family members to connect with their past, release their loved one and prepare to move into the future. I showed up as a compassionate presence of God's abiding love and care while creating a space for the unfolding of a mystery. I advocated for the family and represented the medical institution. I had the privilege to participate in the important work that was completed with honor and devotion. Like the family members, I was transformed by this experience and have moved to a new place in my spiritual journey.

References

Hansberry, J. (RN) (2013). Administrative Director, Swedish Center for Research and Innovation, Swedish Health Services. Personal Communication dated 17 January 2013.

Turner, V. (1967) *The Forest of Symbols*. Ithaca, NY: Cornell University Press.

van Gennep, A. (1961) *The Rites of Passage*. Chicago, IL: University of Chicago Press.

Chapter 14

Critical Response to Palliative Case Studies

A Chaplain's Perspective

David Mitchell

Introduction

Each of these case studies set within the context of palliative care highlights effectively something of 'what chaplains do' and how they think about what they do. To those outside the profession they might seem to be surprising and creative in-depth spiritual encounters; to chaplains they might appear normal: for example, David's story from Old Jerusalem – tragic in its own right but normal in its context. This is by no means to belittle the case studies or their stories but rather to take us beyond the engaging storyline to look beneath for the essence of good chaplaincy care and practice.

In seeking to use these palliative care case studies to identify issues for discussion and debate, it is clear that they work on a number of levels: they can help chaplains engage with the self-awareness of who we are and how that influences our care; they can help us realize the diversity of the role and how it is changing; and they can help us determine what is good practice and realize the importance of reflective practice.

The following sections tease out issues from the case studies and explore the questions these issues might give rise to for individual chaplains and the questions we might engage with as a profession.

Self-awareness

In each of the case studies we get to know something of the chaplains themselves and their religious and spiritual roots; for Chaplains Redl and Weyls these are quite detailed. Do these personal descriptions have a bearing on the case studies? Do they matter to the patients and families? Not really. However, what they do is root the chaplain somewhere and give them a base from which to journey. As spiritual care becomes less mainstream religious and more spiritually diverse, is it important that chaplains be rooted in a mainstream faith community? The question is posed not to protect the rights of mainstream faith communities but to protect and sustain individual chaplains. The UK Board of Healthcare Chaplaincy (UKBHC) recognizes the need for chaplains to have a recognized status within a mainstream faith community or belief group as part of their personal spiritual development (see UKBHC 2014a, 4.2.3).

Self-awareness is the key (Gordon, Kelly and Mitchell 2011). What do chaplains think about life and health, illness, dying and death? How do we balance and integrate the diversity of the care we offer with our own faith and beliefs? Chaplain Weyls' skill in journeying from his roots and balancing the rites of Christian sacraments with traditional Native American death rituals is one example of how this journey of self-awareness can work in practice.

Faith, belief and culture

In each of the three case studies we see faith, belief and culture interwoven into the individual stories of the people for whom care is being given. The religious practices described date back to earlier life experiences, and as death approaches they become more significant. David may have rejected religion as 'bad' and prayer with it; however, for Lee and her father, and for Esmeralda, Maria, Melchior and the family, comfort came in the reassurance of prayer and religious practice. The request for the 'last rites' may be a regular request in palliative care, but to a chaplain it says something more: it speaks of a religion that comes from memory (often childhood) rather than recent practice.

Chaplain Redl, in her reflection on the Middle East and the mix of religion and culture that is part of everyone's lives, suggests people in the Middle East have a stronger background in Christianity, Islam and Judaism; however, this situation is not unique to the Middle East. In Northern Ireland and West Central Scotland the same depth of feeling exists within Christianity, and the Catholic or Protestant division has a similar and heartfelt religious, political and cultural mix: people know what they are and what they are not! Interestingly, one of the identifying factors to distinguish between Protestant and Catholic, and that marks you as one or the other, is how the 'Lord's Prayer' is said (debts or trespasses, and the ascription of glory at the end or not). That same Lord's Prayer that can single people out also brought such comfort to Lee and her father, and to the family gathered around Esmeralda's bed. The challenge for a Christian chaplain might be to consider how we use the Lord's Prayer: Do you stay within your own tradition and in the form you know and use in your faith tradition, or do you use and respect what others would find familiar? Is it a question of integrity of faith, or is it responsive pastoral care?

These three case studies offer very different experiences of faith, belief and culture, and yet they are in many ways ordinary in the world of palliative care chaplaincy. Is seeking to bring meaning at the end of life in a world where communities and families are becoming increasingly diverse in faith, belief and culture the norm or the exception?

The uniqueness of chaplaincy

In the UK throughout the 1990s healthcare chaplaincy set religion aside and sought to help healthcare professionals understand that spirituality was different from religion: a person's spirituality might include religion, but equally it might not. Having won the argument over the broad nature of spirituality, chaplaincy is again reclaiming its religious roots, and in the ever present need to provide evidence-based practice and demonstrate value for money, chaplaincy is rediscovering that its uniqueness is in the understanding and practice of religious care within the context of spiritual care.

On the face of it these case studies demonstrate the importance of healthcare chaplaincy that is underpinned by religious experience and practice. However, what is it that is unique? Is it the different faith communities and belief groups in which the chaplains are rooted? Is it about applying religious ministry in a chaplaincy context? Is it about having a personal rootedness in faith that allows us to understand how faith and belief systems work? Is it about having the confidence to hold together what on the face of it are conflicting traditions yet present together in an individual or family (like Chaplain Weyls did)? Or is the uniqueness in being able to hold all that diversity and variety in our heads and hands, and help it make sense to those for whom we are caring? Add to this mix the question: Can a humanist be a chaplain, and if so, what is their uniqueness? (The old definition of humanists as 'people of no faith' has given way to a more positive definition as a 'belief group' which recognizes a cohesive system of values or beliefs; UKBHC 2014b.)

Communication skills

Core to good spiritual care and palliative care are communication skills (Puchalski 2013; Fallowfield 2010). Each of these case studies has a few sections of verbatim where we are able to see communication skills at work – skills such as reflection, summarizing, clarifying, open questions, picking up cues and silence. Communication is the 'bread and butter' of chaplaincy and is a skill that we can improve with practice. It is clear that the chaplains in the scenarios understand these skills, though it is also clear that self-reflection as we have here can take us only part of the way. When teaching advanced communication skills in a multidisciplinary setting, unlike other healthcare professions, chaplains have inordinate difficulty in describing and role-playing 'what they find difficult' when it is based on actual case scenarios. However, chaplains usually excel when given something new and challenging (real) to role-play. It may be that, as in these case studies, we always have in our head the whole story and how things turned out in the end.

We see examples of how chaplains reflect on their communication skills in these case studies. Chaplain Huth, in his exchanges with Lee, reflects that he might have missed a cue when she mentioned her brother Ed, and on reflection notes he and Chaplain Roberts never did explore that. He wonders if Ed could have been supported more. However, not going down that road with Lee paid dividends. The difficulty with reflection is that it can raise more questions than it answers as we delve into what might have been different. Perhaps we need to do this reflection with others to gain perspective.

There is a stark contrast in the way Chaplains Redl and Weyls use the skill of silence. For Chaplain Redl, it is about patience and presence and creating a safe space. For Chaplain Weyls, it is about awkwardness in waiting, and he seeks to fill the silence with something (the 'Litany of Saints' prayers) – a learning experience for both chaplains. Chaplain Weyls' dilemma, in wanting to fill the silence rather than stay with the awkwardness of the silence, is rooted in complexity. That awkward space of silence was in the midst of a complex scenario that was challenging on so many levels. It takes strength of character to reflect on a complex case and conversation, and again stresses the need for safe and effective reflective practice with others.

Teamwork

The Association of Hospice and Palliative Care Chaplains (AHPCC) lists multidisciplinary teamwork as a required standard and an essential element of palliative care (AHPCC 2006). Peter Speck, a chaplain, devotes a whole book to the topic (Speck 2006). It is interesting that these scenarios do not mention multidisciplinary team working, which raises questions as to whether the chaplains attended or fed into multidisciplinary team meetings; this is unlikely in a busy acute-care setting, such as Chaplain Weyls' hospital, yet more likely an opportunity for Chaplain Redl or Chaplains Huth and Roberts. Were the wider team members aware of the depth of work Chaplains Redl and Huth and Roberts were putting in with their patients? Were they involved and supporting in their own way? Was there a sense of working together? We don't know, and it may have been worth exploring.

The challenge for chaplaincy in teamwork is how to make it work. A stand-alone chaplain or a small team of individuals working part-time may not have an opportunity for multidisciplinary working – time doesn't allow it. Similarly, when facilitating religious care through colleagues from a particular faith community, as in Chaplain Weyls' case, team working brings its own challenges and tensions. Its absence raises questions about chaplaincy and teams. How do chaplains relate to multidisciplinary teams, the wider healthcare team and their chaplaincy team?

Spiritual suffering/pain

Spiritual pain is a widely used term, sometimes referred to as 'total pain'. The term spiritual pain is all too easy to associate with physical pain, and physical pain often has a spiritual root, as in the case of David. The difficulty is that, all too often for the healthcare professionals seeking to alleviate physical pain, the cause might actually be spiritual, and a spiritual cause is often the last resort rather than a consideration from the beginning (Mitchell 2011).

Spiritual pain manifests as suffering. It is hard to define in descriptive terms but we know it when we see it: anxiety; hopelessness; changes in character and demeanor; physical symptoms, such as pain that moves around or is uncontrollable with medication and combined with sleeplessness. David's 'suffering' is a classic example of spiritual suffering/

pain. It is only by Chaplain Redl working in her creative way, through silence, tea and gaining trust, that we get to see and hear David's pain for what it is. However, it is not always that dramatic or clear: Andrew also seems to be experiencing spiritual suffering, which is eased by the reciting of the Lord's Prayer.

The challenge for chaplaincy is how can we raise awareness of spiritual suffering with the wider healthcare team, and move spiritual suffering/pain from its low base of last resort?

Reflective practice

Having identified the issues raised by the case studies, and broached the questions they raise on 'what chaplains do' and 'what they think about what they do', one final area remains: reflective practice. When considering self-awareness of our beliefs and practice, the diversity of faith, belief and culture, our use and development of communication skills, how we relate in teamwork and how we seek to alleviate spiritual suffering, it becomes clear that chaplains are carrying a weight of responsibility and considerable and challenging diversity. What do we do with all that?

Reflective practice is an essential element of chaplaincy practice, not an optional extra. The UKBHC devotes a whole capability to the topic and identifies clear competences for using a structured method of reflective practice: to reflect on case material; to reconcile our personal spirituality with the needs of others; to consider how belief systems interact and relate; and to think about how therapeutic relationships can affect our own beliefs and attitudes (see UKBHC 2014a, 4.1).

Case studies are a valuable tool in reflective practice and provide useful starting points for in-depth study and reflection. Indeed, a recently developed values-based reflective practice model uses a form of case study as an integral part of the practice (Paterson and Kelly 2013).

Case studies as an educational tool

Case studies are a useful tool in highlighting particular issues and themes for discussion and debate. Chaplain Redl's experiences with David could be adapted as a tool for teaching about spiritual pain; Chaplain Weyls' could be adapted as a tool for teaching on faith, belief and culture at the end of life; and Chaplains Huth and Roberts' could be adapted as a tool for teaching on anticipatory grief, family dynamics or pastoral care. The key words in each case are 'could be adapted'. The difficulty with these case studies as they are presented is that they are whole and complete. We have the background of the chaplain, a description of the scenario and encounter, then the analysis, discussion and conclusion. Where else is there to go? Chaplains Huth and Roberts note that their study is but one part of a wider scenario, yet the part we have is complete in itself.

Case studies are a very valuable tool for 'earthing' theory in practice, and are particularly useful for the ethereal topic of spiritual care. However, their value is in the discussion they generate and the individual analysis that follows; they are at their best when they introduce a case scenario and allow people to think, discern and discuss for themselves.

Conclusion

One of the key tasks in professional chaplaincy education is encouraging chaplains to read and present current literature as evidence of their thinking. In theological study, books never date and only add to the depth of the subject. In healthcare study, literature is expected to be current, that is, published in the past 5–10 years. Perhaps a useful question to chaplains could be: If you were to turn to your bookshelves, what is the most current book you have on spiritual care in healthcare?

Since 2008 there has been a marked rise in the number of journal articles and books published by chaplains on the topic of spirituality in healthcare. Why is it that none of this literature appears in the reference lists of these case studies and that, in the main, much of the literature cited dates from 10–40 years ago? This begs the question of how chaplains can be engaged in keeping up to date with the developments in spiritual care and healthcare chaplaincy. Perhaps the answer lies, at least in part, in taking continuing professional development more seriously and making it a requirement for professional registration (Fraser 2013).

References

Association of Hospice and Palliative Care Chaplains (AHPCC) (2006) *Standards for Hospice and Palliative Care Chaplaincy.* Available at www.ukbhc.org. uk/sites/default/files/ahpcc_standards_for_hospice_and_palliative_care_chaplaincy_2006.pdf, accessed on 1 December 2014.

Fallowfield, L. (2010) 'Communication with the patient and the family in palliative medicine.' In G. Hanks, N.I. Cherny, N.A. Christakis, M. Fallon, S. Kaasa and R.K. Portonoy (eds) *Oxford Textbook of Palliative Medicine* (4th edn). Oxford: Oxford University Press, 333–341.

Fraser, D. (2013) 'CPD: An essential component of healthcare chaplaincy.' *Health and Social Care Chaplaincy 1*, 1, 22–34.

Gordon, T., Kelly, E. and Mitchell, D. (2011) *Spiritual Care for Healthcare Professionals: Reflecting on Clinical Practice.* London: Radcliffe.

Mitchell, D. (2011) 'Spiritual and cultural issues at the end of life.' *Medicine 39*, 11, 678–679.

Paterson, M. and Kelly, E. (2013) 'Values-based reflective practice: A method developed in Scotland for spiritual care practitioners.' *Practical Theology 6*, 1, 51–68.

Puchalski, C.M. (2013) 'Restorative medicine.' In M. Cobb, C.M. Puchalski and B. Rumbold (eds) *Oxford Textbook of Spirituality in Healthcare.* Oxford: Oxford University Press, 197–210.

Speck, P. (2006) *Teamwork in Palliative Care: Fulfilling or Frustrating?* Oxford: Oxford University Press.

UK Board of Healthcare Chaplaincy (UKBHC) (2014a) *Spiritual and Religious Care Capabilities and Competences for Healthcare Chaplains Level 5 and 6.* Available at www.ahpcc.org.uk, accessed on 9 January 2014.

UK Board of Healthcare Chaplaincy (UKBHC) (2014b) *Code of Conduct for Healthcare Chaplains.* Available at www.ahpcc.org.uk, accessed on 9 January 2014.

Chapter 15
Critical Response to Palliative Case Studies
A Nurse's Perspective

Barbara Pesut

Dying is hard work for which our healthcare systems are poorly designed. Patients have limited time to live; healthcare providers have limited time to care. This makes for a dynamic fraught with challenges. Conversations about wishes for care are often superficial or absent. Navigating an inefficient system takes up the limited time and energy available to patients and families. Few healthcare providers have the time or preparation to sit with patients and consider the difficult questions that characterize the end of life. Will my being endure? How have I lived my life? How will that influence what comes next?

Here is where chaplains are most visible. The chaplain creates a safe space at the end of life for considering these ultimate questions. In this space, personhood is protected and dignified as the inevitable losses unfold. Chaplains accomplish this work through presence, rituals, prayer, spiritual texts and advocacy (Harper and Rudnick 2010). The palliative care studies presented here provide an intimate look at this care in three diverse scenarios: an elderly veteran with advanced dementia residing in a Canadian publicly funded residential care facility and his caregiver; a middle-aged man with cancer living out his final days in a small hospice-like facility in Jerusalem; and the family of an elderly First Nations woman being taken off life support in a state-of-the-art, not-for-profit hospital in the United States. I will first reflect on each of the cases individually and then make some comments about the essential role of chaplaincy in palliative care.

As I reflect on these case studies, it is important to locate myself as a scholar working in a publicly funded healthcare system, where the role of the chaplain has not been well recognized. I am a nurse who has worked in Canadian healthcare as a practitioner, educator and researcher for over 30 years. My program of research over the past decade has focused on improving end-of-life care for diverse populations. In this research, I have interviewed and shadowed spiritual care providers seeing first-hand the valuable, yet relatively invisible, work they do.

Reflections on the case studies

The case study presented by Chaplains Huth and Roberts addresses one of the most challenging scenarios in maintaining personhood at the end of life: that of dementia. Lee loses her father as she has known him long before his physical death and so is faced with layered and progressive losses. She takes on the difficult task of caregiver and proxy decision maker in isolation after the death of her mother and the estrangement of her brother.

Chaplain Roberts describes the care he provided to create a safe space for Andrew's personhood amidst declining cognitive function. He used familiar rituals and prayers to provide an orienting effect. He provided continuity and companionship that became less verbal, and yet perhaps more present, as Andrew's function declined. His approach was one of calm persistence in light of the potential for dementia-related agitation. Chaplain Roberts' 'thank you' in response to Andrew's sharing of his feeling of the presence of God is a mark of ultimate respect. It beautifully acknowledged the reciprocity that occurs between two individuals who stand together before the presence of God, even when one has declining function. This respect for Andrew's personhood continued beyond death in the celebration of his contributions to life. This is an example of dignity-preserving care in the face of one of life's ultimate indignities.

What is particularly interesting in this case study is the role shared by Chaplains Huth and Roberts as Lee struggles to 'do the right thing'. This is an excellent example of the importance of religious ethics in the context of healthcare and the necessity of having individuals skilled in the negotiation of these ethics. In this case, Lee was struggling under the burden of being the sole decision maker for what were inevitably complex and potentially guilt-ridden decisions. In the past, her father had provided guidance for her life, but the roles were now reversed. She was entrusted with his care and well-being. Drawing upon their Catholic roots, she turned to Chaplain Huth, a Catholic priest, for guidance in doing the right thing. It is interesting to note that despite her established relationship with Chaplain Roberts, it was particularly important for her to have someone who was able to work within her religious tradition to understand the 'good'. In effect, she needed a substitute father to help her grapple with the issues at hand.

Chaplain Huth embodied that same concern for providing a safe space for Lee's personhood. He entered the relationship carefully and sensitively, allowing Lee to take the lead. He waited for her to disclose what she felt he may have disapproved of, and then he skillfully used humor to set her at ease. For example, when she disclosed that she was a hippie (and by implication rebellious to the church), with laughter he suggested that perhaps she was the 'first hippie in Canada'. He was telling her that she was not alone – many others have been there too. He helped her to articulate her challenges and provided a safe space for her to reflect on those challenges. He instructed her in the rituals according to the Catholic tradition. He helped her to identify areas of strength, including the pride her parents had in her, as a basis upon which to go forward and have confidence in her decisions. In essence, Chaplain Huth helped Lee to construct a 'good' that she knew would be in keeping with her father's own wishes if he had had the capacity to make his own decisions. This is the ideal of substitute decision making.

Two questions arise for me in this scenario. The first question relates to Lee's suffering over how such a good man could die in such a difficult way. This is a common struggle for people of faith, and it is interesting to me that this particular point of Lee's suffering was not pursued. Furthermore, there was little discussion about the decisions Lee was being asked to make. Her comments that she was driving the doctor crazy with questions, and her struggles over whether she has done everything possible, are a sign that perhaps there was more to be understood in terms of making 'good' decisions. Was she being asked to remove treatment? Here is where it is so essential for spiritual care providers to have palliative care knowledge and to be connected to the team so that they can help family members wrestle with the good in a more concrete way.

Chaplain Redl's case study is interesting because, despite the overarching dictate of chaplaincy to 'meet individuals at the point of their perceived need' (Harper and Rudnick 2010, p.199), in this exemplar initially only Chaplain Redl perceives that need. What is even more intriguing about this case study is the intersectionality of class, culture and religion. Chaplain Redl and the recipient of care, David, are opposites. Chaplain Redl is a conservative rabbi, raised in Germany, with a background in nursing and chaplaincy and a strong orientation toward social justice. Each of these identities has the potential to position her favorably or unfavorably depending upon the recipient of care. David, although described as an Orthodox Jew, is an example of the diverse melding of culture and religion that is so indicative of the modern world. He had Jewish, Christian and Muslim friends, and spoke three languages fluently. Their temperaments are also polarized. Chaplain Redl is a study in quiet patience and perseverance as she seeks to create a safe space for David to engage. She is a watcher who studies David and adapts her approach accordingly. Her only challenging statement occurs when she seeks to connect with him. In response to his claim that he doesn't like to talk to people, she somewhat cheekily replies that he shouts just fine and speaks loudly through his actions. David, on the other hand, is a study in passion – angry outbursts, humor, childlike joy and fierce belligerence. He is a doer, engaged in all aspects of his care. She *reflects* on her feelings; he *expresses* his feelings. And yet, they still manage to come together in a healing relationship.

Chaplain Redl facilitated a unique healing whereby David's existential pain was reduced and he was better able to connect with others. How was she able to do this? What stands out from the case study is her remarkable reflexivity. She evaluated her own needs in relation to his. She worked tirelessly to see between the lines of the encounters. A stellar example is her understanding that although he had experienced deep trauma, that trauma was eclipsed by the social upheaval that had characterized life in Jerusalem, leaving him without the ability to have his unique trauma legitimized. This case study describes the quintessential outcome for chaplaincy in palliative care – a peaceful, connected death.

There is a puzzling element to this case study. Chaplain Redl describes David as both childlike in his humor and joy, and broken in his anger and alienation. She saw that David's anger and alienation was reduced, and that he felt the presence of God over his final days, but still she questioned whether she could have connected him better to God. In other words, even though Chaplain Redl saw the Godlike qualities within him throughout their encounters, she still wondered about the connection. One can't help but wonder if there was more reciprocity in this relationship than is discussed in the narrative. Perhaps, while Chaplain Redl helped David to connect with persons, David helped her to see that God's connection is enduring and particularly strong within those who have suffered deeply, despite outward appearances.

The story of Chaplain Weyls, Maria and her family brings to mind a spiritual broker. In healthcare, we use knowledge brokers to bridge the gaps between research and practice. In similar fashion, Chaplain Weyls used religious, spiritual and healthcare knowledge to bridge the worlds of Catholicism and Native American spirituality, families and healthcare providers, institutional policies and spiritual rituals, and of his own location and the needs of others. This was all the more skillful in light of the fact that Chaplain Weyls did not have the luxury of a long-term relationship with this family. Entering the world of the dying at times such as this requires a particularly sophisticated approach; he describes it as becoming a student, companion and privileged participant. The exemplar is full of rich narratives that illustrate how Chaplain Weyls enacts these roles. What further stands out in this case study is how Chaplain Weyls' sacramental and incarnational theology allows him to enter so many diverse realms with confidence. He sees God as present in all circumstances and seeks to be the host of that mystery.

In the telling of this story, Chaplain Weyls speaks twice about his own grief in the loss of his identity as a Roman Catholic priest. I cannot help but wish he had reflected more on that in relation to this case. Beyond the limitations of not being able to fulfill the sacramental role, I suspect that it may have been the loss of this identity that enabled him to adopt new ones that bridged so many worlds so skillfully. Explicating this transition more would be a valuable teaching moment for other chaplains encountering similar losses.

Reflections on the role of chaplaincy in palliative care

As I pondered these case studies, I could not help but think of liminal spaces – those spaces in which we wait, leaving the old but not yet settling into the new. Palliative patients exist in liminal spaces. Chaplains wait with them in those spaces. The profession of chaplaincy occupies a liminal space in many countries, particularly those that are grappling with the role of religion in publicly funded healthcare. Chaplaincy services are typically the first to go when healthcare budgets become tight. Now is the time to articulate the contribution that chaplains make to palliative care and to argue a compelling case for why their role is so essential at this juncture in history.

The case studies presented here provide important insights into the contributions of chaplains. The power of story is remarkable. Tacit knowledge is revealed and contributions to care are made visible. How outcomes are achieved and the philosophies that support those outcomes are illuminated. As I reflect on the language used and the stories told, three things stand out. First is the dignity and respect for personhood. The intrinsic worth of patients and families is threaded throughout each exemplar. In a healthcare culture that struggles to integrate a patient-centered approach, and in a cultural milieu that has adopted an instrumental approach to spirituality, this perspective is remarkably refreshing. Second is the importance of chaplains having palliative- and healthcare-specific knowledge (Puchalski *et al.* 2009). It seems to me that one cannot fully understand the issues that patients and families are facing unless one has some baseline healthcare knowledge about the context. Third is the emphasis on feelings. I wondered about this approach. I have argued within nursing literature that overemphasis on positive emotions may not do justice to the spiritual journey of suffering; indeed, it may inadvertently stigmatize those who are suffering (Pesut *et al.* 2008). As I revisited the chaplaincy literature in preparing for this response, I saw aspirations for outcomes of meaningful connections, peace, healing, control, hope and the management of negative emotions (Harper and Rudnick 2010). In light of these aspirations, the focus on feelings as tangible outcomes is understandable. Positive emotions were realized in each of these exemplars, but I was left wondering how one might gauge the effectiveness of care *without* positive emotions. Are there essential contributions that chaplains make to care that do not rest upon such laudable goals, and how does one maintain meaning in one's work if these goals cannot be achieved?

The chaplain in modern healthcare serves as a religious and spiritual navigator in a way that no one else can. In a study we conducted that explored the negotiation of religious and spiritual plurality in healthcare, chaplains were the only healthcare providers who consistently had the competence to bridge diversity while continuing to deepen understanding within their own religious traditions (Pesut *et al.* 2012). In palliative care there is a dawning realization that early conversations around goals of care are critical. Without such conversations, no healthcare system will be sustainable in light of a population aging with complex chronic illness. Chaplains understand the nature and power of religious ethics in these decisions. Chaplain Huth worked with Lee to help her identify what was right for her to do in the context of her father's religious faith. Ideally, Chaplain Huth would have been part of the team deliberations so that he could have communicated this knowledge to healthcare providers, who all too often dismiss religious ethics as irrelevant to modern care. Furthermore, high-quality palliative care supports the rituals of passage from this life into the next. Chaplains have the knowledge and skills to navigate the 'super-nova' of spiritualities (Taylor 2007, p.300) that have resulted from the melding of religious traditions. Like Chaplain Weyls, they negotiate a hospitable space that respects the safety of patients, families and staff. Finally, high-quality palliative care pays attention to those on the margins. Once designed as poorhouses, hospitals remain places where there is overrepresentation of those most vulnerable in society. Yet the system does not have the capacity to care for those whose healing is not primarily found in the physical domain. Like Chaplain Redl and Chaplain Roberts, chaplains provide a supportive presence for those for whom personhood is at risk. Chaplains have an essential role to play in the delivery of palliative care. Case studies such as these reveal the nuanced way in which chaplains perform care, thus building credibility for the profession and helping to prepare the next generation of chaplains.

References

Harper, J.M. and Rudnick, J.E. (2010) 'The role of the chaplain in palliative care.' In G. Hanks, N.I. Cherny, N.A. Christakis, M. Fallon, S. Kaasa and R.K. Portonoy (eds) *Oxford Textbook of Palliative Medicine* (4th edn). Oxford: Oxford University Press, 197–205.

Pesut, B., Fowler, M., Johnston Taylor, E., Reimer-Kirkham, S. and Sawatzky, R. (2008) 'Conceptualizing spirituality and religion for healthcare.' *Journal of Clinical Nursing 17*, 21. Available at www.ncbi.nlm.nih.gov/pubmed/18665876, accessed 1 October 2013.

Pesut, B., Reimer-Kirkham, S., Sawatzky, R., Woodland, G. and Peverall, P. (2012) 'Hospitable hospitals in a diverse society: from chaplains to spiritual care providers.' *Journal of Religion and Health 51*, 3, 825–836.

Puchalski, C.M., Ferrell, B., Virani, R., Otis-Green, S., et al. (2009) 'Improving the quality of spiritual care as a dimension of palliative care: The report of the consensus conference.' *Journal of Palliative Medicine 12*, 10, 885–904.

Taylor, C. (2007) *A Secular Age*. Cambridge, MA: Belknap Press of Harvard University Press.

Part 4
Ethical Concerns

Chapter 16

Ethical Issues in
Case Study Publication

David B. McCurdy

Introduction

My task in this chapter is to comment on a limited yet important aspect of the case study process: the ethical concerns that arise in preparing to publish chaplaincy case studies. From one perspective, this chapter is a sequel to a longer journal article on ethical concerns in case study publication (McCurdy and Fitchett 2011). It seeks, in part, to distill the findings of that earlier article and make them more accessible to chaplains and other interested parties. (Readers can refer to that article for more extended analysis of some issues discussed here.) This chapter also draws on the case studies in this volume to elaborate themes from the earlier article that merit further attention or appear in new forms here. Finally, I suggest additional ethical concerns or directions that seem to emerge from these case studies.

The focus on the ethics of case study publication is a relatively narrow one. As such, it can be distinguished from ethical concerns that arise in chaplains' practice or reflection on practice in these cases. For example, Zollfrank explicitly identifies an 'ethical dilemma' presented by her inclination to suggest an alternative religious/spiritual framework to a young gay man from a Roman Catholic background in a highly communal Hispanic culture. This issue and other questions of ethical chaplaincy practice, suggested by these case studies and others, may deserve focused consideration in future case study-related publications.

The ethical landscape

The entrée to ethical awareness in chaplaincy case study publication is most often the question of obtaining permission or consent to publish the case (Fitchett 2011). For chaplains, this concern is not just theoretical – it nags at the conscientious chaplain who desires above all to respect and protect the spiritual care relationship yet also seeks to improve chaplaincy practice and advance the spiritual care field. In a previous case study project involving oncology chaplains, Fitchett (2011) mined the psychology case study literature and worked with the chaplains to develop an approach to the permission issue. In gathering case material for the present volume, editors Fitchett and Nolan built on that approach and also invited case study authors to draw on McCurdy and Fitchett (2011) in considering permission-related issues.

While permission to publish is typically the presenting ethical issue in case study publication, upon examination the permission question exposes a number of underlying ethical concerns. Perhaps the most obvious concern is the question of preserving confidentiality and privacy. The very notion of 'publication' seems to contradict the foundation of practice in spiritual care, as it does in related fields such as psychotherapy. Confidentiality, which can be viewed as an aspect of 'informational privacy' (Beauchamp and Childress 2013, p.316), is deemed essential to the trust that patients and clients place in their chaplain- and therapist-confidants and to the benefits they hope to derive from these relationships. In this view, confidentiality serves utilitarian purposes: all parties, including both current and future patients and providers, are thought to be best served if confidentiality is maintained. At the same time, patient autonomy, understood not as a mere abstraction but as a person's moral right to have some control over information concerning himself or herself, is respected by confidential practice.

Normally, in the healthcare setting, the circle of confidentiality expands to encompass the 'team' involved in providing care to the patient and family (Loewy and Loewy 2007, p.53). As members of the team, chaplains also share with other team members information deemed relevant to the patient's care and the team's goals (McCurdy 2012). On the other hand, in the religious or spiritual sphere, and perhaps especially among Christians, adherence to confidentiality has typically been viewed as sacrosanct, indeed as 'secret keeping' (Blodgett 2008, p.33). Arguably, healthcare chaplains, at least those from the Christian tradition, are influenced by both understandings of confidentiality (McCurdy and Fitchett 2011; McCurdy 2012). In practice, however, the healthcare norm with its wider circle of 'confidants' tends to predominate, as exemplified by several of the cases in this collection (e.g. Grossoehme, Zollfrank) – though perhaps not all (e.g. Swift).

When it comes to publication and permission to publish, ethical and religious concerns about confidentiality are joined, and sometimes intensified, by legal or regulatory concerns. In the US context, an existing ethical and legal focus on confidentiality was amplified by the federal Health Insurance Portability and Accountability Act (HIPAA) regulations in 2003. The HIPAA Privacy Rule sets out the ways in which the 'privacy' of health information is to be preserved and specifies when and to whom such information may be disclosed (Office for Civil Rights 2003). In reality, compliance with the Privacy Rule *as regulation* in publishing case study material is a relatively straightforward matter; like some other regulations, it has engendered more compliance anxiety than may be warranted. Its *ethical intent*, namely, drawing attention to the sensitivity of and need to protect a broad range of information about persons, can be a helpful reminder in the process of disguising information about case study subjects.

The deliberate use here of the term 'subjects' provides an entry point to a second legal and regulatory concern associated with the permission question, namely, whether case studies are research. Labeling case reports 'studies' suggests, at least in the US, the question of whether these studies should be considered 'research', that is, subject to federal regulations governing research. If so, the case studies would be subject to oversight by local institutional review boards (IRBs), usually under the aegis of the healthcare institutions where the case studies are based. While the 'research' question is posed in bureaucratic terms, the underlying concern is, again, an ethical one. Human subjects of research are generally considered to be in a vulnerable position, usually exposed to some form and level of risk, and both in need of and deserving of protection because their participation in research contributes to the greater good.

On the regulatory front, unanimous IRB advice in the earlier oncology project was that single case studies lacked an overarching research design and were therefore not research in the regulatory sense and so did not require IRB oversight (McCurdy and Fitchett 2011, p.63). This was true even if there was intent to publish the case studies (McCurdy and Fitchett 2011). In practice, this meant that obtaining informed consent for publication – a more complex and demanding standard than obtaining permission – was unnecessary. (This determination did not release case study authors from the need to observe applicable HIPAA constraints on the disclosure of personally identifying information.) Even so, consideration of the research question highlighted parallels that could not be ignored between case study and research. The parallels involve both risk and intent. Case study publication, even when using pseudonyms and altering personal details, inevitably involves some level of risk that case study subjects' identities will be discovered (Gavey and Braun 1997). The probability of discovery may be quite small, but the consequences of discovery may include psychological, spiritual, relational and even financial harms (Gavey and Braun 1997; Miller 2004; McCurdy and Fitchett 2011). Moreover, like published research, chaplaincy case studies are not published for the benefit of the patient (or other participants in the case), but for other purposes.

What can justify exposing patients or others to such risks, however improbable? We concluded that the intent to promote 'humane' aims – benefiting future patients and recipients of spiritual care and improving chaplaincy practice – could justify publication, even when professionally self-interested aims, such as advancing the standing of the field, are also involved (McCurdy and Fitchett 2011, p.65). However, the dual reality of risk and non-therapeutic intent seem to make the term 'case study *subject*' an appropriate way to frame what these case study participants are asked to agree to. The fact that some participants appreciate being subjects of publication may be a secondary benefit to them (e.g. in Grossoehme's case; Cooper 2011) but does not obviate the cautionary considerations noted here; nor does the possibility that some subjects might agree to publication without knowing or caring about its specific purpose. A patient's autonomous permission or consent, in other words, is not by itself a sufficient justification for the risks of publication (McCurdy and Fitchett 2011).

Specific concerns

A number of lingering questions and potential avenues for further ethical inquiry emerged from the earlier oncology case study project (McCurdy and Fitchett 2011). The cases and reflections appearing in the current collection suggest that our earlier set of concerns might be refined and recast under three main headings: (1) permission/consent; (2) protecting identity and confidentiality; and (3) respect for non-primary case participants. Within these categories there will be a discussion of subordinate concerns, such as the timing of permission requests or the non-availability of the primary subject to give permission, that were also highlighted in the prior article.

First, however, a word about two important topics that do not appear under the three main headings is necessary. After the oncology chaplaincy project, it appeared that the question of whether case study should be considered 'research', at least in the formal US regulatory sense, was largely settled (McCurdy and Fitchett 2011). The current set of cases essentially confirms that conclusion. However, it remains wise for chaplains to consult their local IRB or an equivalent body regarding plans for case study publication (McCurdy and Fitchett 2011). It should also be recalled that the research question mattered in part because of its association with the question of obtaining not mere permission to publish but formal consent, akin to consent to participate in research. (That question receives further attention in the section on permission/consent.)

Our earlier reasoning and conclusions (McCurdy and Fitchett 2011), discussed above, about what could justify risks to subjects in case study publication still seem sound. As a result of reading the cases collected here, I later suggest an additional reason to support, and indeed promote, case study publication.

Permission/consent

We (McCurdy and Fitchett 2011) have advocated obtaining permission to publish from the patient whenever possible or feasible. The range of cases in this collection suggests augmenting that recommendation to encompass permission from the patient or another focal case study subject, such as Lee (the patient's daughter) in Huth and Roberts' case, and certainly a parent or other surrogate when the patient is a minor. In addition, seeking the assent of the minor patient with some maturity seems a best practice and perhaps obligatory (e.g. in Grossoehme's case). These patients are certainly not 'little adults', as Grossoehme states, and others must give permission on their behalf, yet they are not 'mere children' either.

We have also suggested that obtaining permission from family members when the patient is deceased or unavailable to give permission is a 'gold standard' for practice (McCurdy and Fitchett 2011, p.71). In the case by Huth and Roberts, the permission given by Lee, the patient's daughter, effectively served as permission on both her and her deceased father's behalf. In some cases, however, chaplain sensitivity to people and circumstances, plus consultation from colleagues and/or institutional authorization when feasible, may suggest that careful disguise will need to suffice.

Most of the case reports say something about whether and how the author(s) obtained some form of authorization to publish the case. It is striking that the basic issue of obtaining permission is dealt with so variably. In only two of the nine cases is actual permission (plus assent, in one instance) obtained from the patient or a close relative. One case depicts an apparently careful and thought-out process for seeking permission. Others note, apparently quite reasonably, the difficulty or impossibility of obtaining permission from the patient or others and typically describe an alternative institutional process of authorization to publish. Still others do not even mention the issue of obtaining permission, although they may describe other processes for authorizing publication.

Since the editors and the publisher addressed this issue in explicit ways prior to publication, one may imagine that more went on behind the scenes in terms of seeking permission or other authorization than is apparent in some of the case reports. The fact that a number of the case studies were written years after the events of the case may play a role. One could nonetheless wish for more consistent and complete attention to these questions in future case study writing. It could, I think, be viewed as a significant, and standard, element of the 'data' to be developed through a body of case studies.

In particular, the field would benefit from relatively detailed descriptions, such as Grossoehme (in the present book) and Cooper (2011) provide, of how and in what circumstances chaplains broach the subject of permission with case study subjects. In this collection, it would be interesting to know how psychiatric patient Nate's chaplain (in Zollfrank's case) thought about the permission issue in light of Nate's strong fear about losing confidentiality during hospitalization, given that publication may be perceived to pose a significant threat to confidentiality.

Several of the more nitty-gritty permission-related issues that we (McCurdy and Fitchett 2011) considered surface in these cases. One issue is the timing of requests for permission. Envisioning that cases would normally be completed and submitted for publication after the primary chaplaincy relationship ends, and respecting the desire not to complicate that relationship with the specter of publication, we recommended that permission requests be made late in the spiritual care engagement. The pediatric case of LeeAnn (Grossoehme's case), depicting an early stage of a potential long-term relationship with a chronically ill patient, is a reminder that different scenarios are possible. The chaplain's seemingly artful management of requests for assent and permission (met by the patient's and family's apparent equanimity about this prospect) demonstrates that it is possible to accomplish this task in an ongoing relationship, and even to make it part of the spiritual care.

We (McCurdy and Fitchett 2011) also considered the question of written versus verbal permission and, deferring to the diversity of practices that seem to exist, did not recommend a preferred practice. Inevitably, this question partakes of the wider issue of 'permission' versus 'consent'. Formal written permission tends to be thought of as 'consent' whether or not it is actually 'informed' consent with all that term implies in the therapeutic or research context. The more important question would seem to be how much and what kind of information should be provided in the request for permission. We suggested that respect for patients and others *as subjects* may require more than simply asking for their 'yes' to publish. In seeking permission, it seems advisable to note that there is no ironclad guarantee of confidentiality, even with best efforts at disguise and even though the risk should be very low. As a practical matter, asking chaplains, who may already be a bit uneasy about 'making the ask', to be this explicit in cautioning the patient may be expecting a lot. It was not apparent in the accounts here whether chaplains broached this issue when they sought permission.

One apparent new wrinkle in the permission process that emerged here was the way in which some chaplains offered patients and other subjects an opportunity to read the case before publication. We (McCurdy and Fitchett 2011) had framed this option as a way to give subjects input on, and thus some control over, how their identities and personal information are disguised. In the cases at hand, the review option seemed to function more like phase two of a continuing process of granting permission to publish. Twelve-year-old LeeAnn, for example, was told explicitly that she could veto 'presentation' of the case after she read it if she wished, and could comment on the case. Lee (in Huth and Roberts' case), the patient-resident's daughter in a palliative care case, had an opportunity to read the case and comment on it for publication, again not in a context that suggested an emphasis on disguising her identity or others' identities. Still, protecting personal identity and confidential information was a substantial concern and aim in all the case studies.

Protecting identity and confidentiality

Disguising the identity of case study subjects is a *sine qua non* of case study practice. Disguising identity should not be treated as an alternative to seeking permission, but rather as a companion practice to obtaining permission whenever reasonably possible. In any event, chaplains should strive to avoid having 'the identity of, or [confidential] information about, patients in their spiritual care...become known as a result of publication' (McCurdy and Fitchett 2011, p.68).

Whatever approach the chaplains in these case studies took to the permission issue, without exception they disguised the identity of case study participants by using pseudonyms and altering demographic information and/or other potentially identifying details. The problem that chaplains face in disguising subjects' identities is striking a balance between adequate concealment and sufficient disclosure of relevant information to convey the nature and power of the interaction. If a well-disguised case study is rightly described as, in a certain sense, 'based on' what actually happened (e.g. in Piderman's case), authors must also take care not to distort relevant information and inadvertently mislead readers.

The case studies here give little indication of how this process played out in the chaplains' thinking and the decisions they made as they wrote the case. To some extent this seems unavoidable, as describing too fully how one disguised the case runs the risk of unmasking the disguise itself. Even so, the literature in psychology suggests a taxonomy of case disguise 'strategies' (McCurdy and Fitchett 2011, p.68; APA 2010). It should be possible for future chaplain authors to provide somewhat more detail about the kinds of strategies they use.

What some authors did describe, perhaps following guidance offered by the editors, was a process by which they obtained feedback on the adequacy of the disguise. It may be imagined that the review invited by Grossoehme, and perhaps by Huth and Roberts, included a request for such feedback from the subject-readers of their cases. Grossoehme had previously explicitly invited the pediatric patient to select her own pseudonym. Hildebrand, who sought without success to contact the focal case study subject, shared the disguised case report with a hospital social worker who was currently working with the subject. Arguably, the social worker who had knowledge of the subject served as a proxy reviewer, in a sense standing in for the subject herself.

Respect for non-primary case participants

The active efforts made by all authors to protect the primary case study subjects from harms of publication, and by several to ascertain and respect these subjects' wishes regarding publication, reflect a commitment to the well-being and autonomy of patients and other focal subjects. Usually there are other participants who also play a larger or smaller part in a case study; these normally include family members in particular, but the list may extend in a given case to various professionals and others involved in the care process. How should the chaplain author regard them and their role in the case study? Should they, or should some of them, be informed of the case study's publication, asked for permission in advance and perhaps invited to view or review the finished product?

There seems to be no simple and obvious answer to such questions. Inviting all the non-primary case participants, or some but not others, to give permission for publication and/or to review the case seems impractical and might create more relational problems than it would solve. A basic norm does suggest itself, however: the non-primary participants in case study – like the primary subjects – are 'worthy of respect' and deserve to be treated accordingly (McCurdy and Fitchett 2011, p.71). Even unknowingly, they too make a contribution to the potential improvement of spiritual care and well-being of future recipients of spiritual care.

The concrete meaning of a norm of respect for non-primary participants would need to be elucidated over time. To begin with, it seems to suggest that chaplains should develop ways to acknowledge these subjects' anonymous contributions (McCurdy and Fitchett 2011), perhaps with a gesture as simple as a note of acknowledgement at the end of a case. It would also seem that information about them should be subject to the same care for identity protection as would be given to the primary case study subjects.

The norm of respect for these study participants may have other implications beyond questions of permission, grateful acknowledgment or disguising identity. In the current collection, some cases raise ethical questions in the way authors discuss and describe non-primary case participants. In one instance (Huth and Roberts' case) a family member – the patient's son and focal subject's brother, Ed – is ultimately portrayed as a family member who has chosen to distance himself from the family. This characterization appears to come first from the patient and his daughter. Initially, the authors report it as an 'according to her' (the daughter's) characterization, but later the authors themselves refer to 'the emotional distance that Ed put between himself and the rest of the family', implying that indeed Ed was the agent and initiator. While in their reflections they question their ministry to Ed, they do not question the portrait of him as a family culprit.

In the absence of an account by the authors that they had other evidence that Ed had acted to create emotional distance and was wholly responsible for it, one question this account raises is whether, in a study for publication, it is appropriate to describe a participant in this way solely on the basis of others' account of him. The parallel practice question might be whether the chaplains uncritically adopted or overidentified with other family members' point of view about Ed; that question is nonetheless distinct from the question of how Ed is, or should be, characterized in the published case study.

One might argue that this is literally a matter of no consequence to Ed; he will never know what is said about him, nor will others, since the case is 'anonymized'. In other words, especially given the low risk of discovery, he will suffer no harm from the study's references to him. In this instance, two responses may be given. First, it is widely accepted that people – even anonymized people – can be wronged even though they suffer no tangible harm (Beauchamp and Childress 2013). Second, in this instance it is possible that some harm may be done. Ed's sister was given an opportunity to read a draft of the case; she would have seen what the authors said about her brother and his distancing behavior, and might have noted that their comments seem to affirm her 'side' in the family dynamic. Conceivably, she could even say something to her brother about this aspect of the case study. In the end, it seems that some form or forms of injustice may be done to Ed, not through pastoral practice but through pastoral publication.

In another case (Swift's case), a psychiatric patient tells the chaplain that she overheard nursing staff members laughing disparagingly about her, ostensibly because they had learned of her love for another woman now dead. In the case analysis, the chaplain seems to accept what may be only the patient's inference – were they really laughing at her, or for that reason? – without apparent question or independent verification. The chaplain then comments critically about the nursing staff's 'mocking' of the patient and links the 20-year-old case incident to generalizations from a contemporary national report critical of UK nurses' treatment of patients (Hayter 2013). Here the issue is likely not one of harm to the staff – the events are long past and the hospital is not identified – but perhaps there are still questions of fairness in portrayal and assessment and of how to show authorial respect for staff members who, by being discussed, became unknowing contributors to this effort to advance practice in spiritual care.

Clearly there is more to be learned about what it means to respect all case participants in publishing case studies. Identifying some general ways in which respect may be shown to non-primary subjects or groups seems a significant first step. Articulating how such respect is best shown in particular situations will continue to be an opportunity and challenge as new cases are written.

Further comments and future directions

Reflection on these cases suggests several additional areas that may deserve future consideration. I will comment on two areas, in particular, that I believe have implications for future case study work.

Understanding the importance of consultation and authorization

Early on, this volume's editors recommended that case study authors not make certain key decisions on their own but seek consultation and engage in dialogue with colleagues across disciplines. Consultation was recommended especially when a chaplain had a question about whether to obtain permission, how to disguise a case or whether to publish the case. It seems important that the editors emphasized the value of consultation and what I would call external validation. Moreover, in various ways the authors gave evidence of doing something along the lines the editors suggested. Hildebrand, for example, brought together the institutional leaders who initially authorized her case study project plus a senior ethicist to assist her with questions about permission and other issues. Perhaps not incidentally, she had earlier followed editorial guidance by accessing literature on the ethics of publication. Because the chaplain was finally unable to obtain the focal subject's permission, one might say that this consultative arrangement came to double as institutional authorization of the case study's publication.

The reality of institutional authorization and chaplains' recognition that it was needed, especially in the absence of a subject's or surrogate's permission, was in fact a common feature of most of the cases. The form or locus of authorization varied. In one instance it was the IRB, even though the case study was not deemed 'research' (Weyls' case), that seemed indirectly to authorize the publication by giving guidance on what was 'required' to complete it. In other instances, the mere fact that the IRB confirmed that a case study was not research seemed to function *de facto* as institutional authorization to proceed, at least as the chaplains interpreted it. In still other cases it was an administrator or simply 'the institution' that was said to approve or authorize publication and, often, delineated conditions to be met in the prepublication process.

It is noteworthy, on the consultation front, that two of the cases mention consulting the literature about some ethical aspect of publication. One of them modeled his turn to pre-publication patient review and comment on the approach of an earlier chaplain author (Grossoehme, citing Risk 2013).

The aim here is not merely to describe how chaplains used or approached consultation and authorization, but to suggest that the moral significance of these activities merits exploration. One construal might begin with chaplains' sense of responsibility for the welfare of people in their care and simultaneous responsibility to the field in which they practice. Given the fact of this dual responsibility, perhaps chaplains recognized a need for *moral* support as they negotiated ambiguous publication issues that had consequences both for others and for them.

With regard to seeking institutional authorization, one might speculate that this need went beyond the obvious fact that some institutions had ways of doing things that demanded conformity. It may also derive from the reality that publication issues, however mundane they might seem, cannot be neatly separated from the chaplains' spiritual care relationships with the case study subjects. Perhaps, as they felt the weight of their responsibility in and for these relationships, moral support and guidance from other professionals, and even from institutions, might be a source of real help. Whatever the merit of this speculation, future reflection on the ethics of case study publication might do well to examine more closely the dynamics and the meaning of institutional authorization in the case study process. It could be important to hear more from chaplains on how they experience and think through these issues.

At the same time, it can be noted that some chaplains made no discernible reference either to consultation or to institutional authorization in the absence of pre-publication subject or surrogate permission. It is possible that they did not describe all the steps they actually took in this regard. The point is not to call into question the prepublication practices of chaplains who may not have sought consultation and/or authorization before publication. What may be more important at this stage of case study development is to learn how chaplains think through whatever approach they eventually take.

A duty to share

Near the end of a programmatic article on case study publication, Fitchett recounts a chaplain's comment about role-playing a chaplaincy verbatim before a multidisciplinary group: 'We brought down the house because it was like they never…experienced a chaplain's visit before', the chaplain concluded (Lyndes *et al.* 2008, p.74). There are cases here that bring down the house. They do more than 'teach'; they edify. They do more than show chaplains at work, or demonstrate their value as professionals to those willing to pay attention; they open the door to wonder. They begin to expose the mystery of what can happen for good between and within people, seemingly against all odds, in the midst of tragedy, pain and loss. And this does not happen only when the chaplain is at her or his most 'competent'. The cases point to the mystery and hope of what can happen in the relational space between chaplains and those for whom they care. Expertise helps, but the cases also show how expertise must be met by what some would call grace.

In light of this reality, I want to suggest that chaplains' responsibility to write and publish case studies is more than a responsibility to advance a field seeking to survive in difficult times, or a responsibility to improve practice, or even a responsibility to help provide better care to future care recipients. It is also a responsibility to share with the widest possible audience the emotional and spiritual impact of human encounters like those described and reflected on in this book. Whatever spirit or Spirit is at work in these relational spaces needs to be unveiled, at least for a moment, to an audience beyond those in the chaplaincy guild or even the relatively small world of healthcare. Chaplains, I am suggesting, have a duty to share this spirit or Spirit and these experiences, perhaps a duty of a certain evangelism on behalf of this spirit or Spirit and on behalf of the kind of care that helps make its emergence possible. Let the writing and publishing continue, and multiply, with this duty, too, in mind.

References

American Psychological Association (APA) (2010) *Ethical Principles of Psychologists and Codes of Conduct with the 2010 Amendments*. Available at www.apa.org/ethics/code/index.aspx, accessed on 4 July 2014.

Beauchamp, T.L. and Childress, J.F. (2013) *Principles of Biomedical Ethics* (7th edn). Oxford: Oxford University Press.

Blodgett, B.J. (2008) *Lives Entrusted: An Ethic of Trust for Ministry*. Minneapolis, MN: Fortress Press.

Cooper, R.S. (2011) 'Case study of a chaplain's spiritual care for a patient with advanced metastatic breast cancer.' *Journal of Health Care Chaplaincy 17*, 1, 19–37.

Fitchett, G. (2011) 'Making our case(s).' *Journal of Health Care Chaplaincy 17*, 1–2, 3–18.

Gavey, N. and Braun, V. (1997) 'Ethics and the publication of clinical case material.' *Professional Psychology: Research and Practice 28*, 4, 399–404.

Hayter, M. (2013) 'The UK Francis Report: The key messages for nursing.' *Journal of Advanced Nursing 69*, 8, 1–3.

Loewy, R.S. and Loewy, E. (2007) 'Healthcare and the hospital chaplain.' *Medscape General Medicine 9*, 1, 53. Available at www.ncbi.nlm.nih.gov/pmc/articles/ PMC1924976/#__ffn_sectitle, accessed on 4 July 2014.

Lyndes, K.A., Fitchett, G., Thomason, C.L., Berlinger, N. and Jacobs, M.R. (2008) 'Chaplains and quality improvement: Can we make our case by improving our care?' *Journal of Health Care Chaplaincy 15*, 2, 65–79.

McCurdy, D.B. (2012) 'Chaplains, confidentiality and the chart.' *Chaplaincy Today 28*, 2, 20–31.

McCurdy, D.B. and Fitchett, G. (2011) 'Ethical issues in case study publication: "Making our case(s)" ethically.' *Journal of Health Care Chaplaincy 17*, 1–2, 55–74.

Miller, R.B. (2004) *Facing Human Suffering: Psychology and Psychotherapy as Moral Engagement.* Washington, DC: American Psychological Association.

Office for Civil Rights, U.S. Department of Health and Human Services (2003) 'Summary of the HIPAA Privacy Rule.' Available at www.hhs.gov/ocr/privacy/ hipaa/understanding/summary, accessed 2 October 2014.

Risk, J.L. (2013) 'Building a new life: A chaplain's theory based case study of chronic illness.' *Journal of Health Care Chaplaincy 19*, 3, 81–98.

Afterword

John Swinton

Chaplaincy case studies and the refreshing of the healthcare imagination

It has been a pleasure to have been given the opportunity to spend time dwelling in the richness of the case studies presented in this book. I have been challenged, touched and moved by the power and the honesty of the stories and perspectives that have been opened up by the chaplains, and by the thoughtfulness of the responders who, while honest and critical, remain respectful and hospitable. The book is truly critical and conversational in the best way that such terms should be used. In this brief Afterword I simply want to reflect on the concept of case studies and the possibilities that this approach has for enabling imaginative, creative and authentically healing chaplaincy practices.

Rejuvenating the healthcare imagination

Good healthcare chaplaincy requires a certain kind of imagination. It is easy to overlook the fact that imagination is vital for the ways in which we explain and negotiate the world and conceptualize, plan and carry out healthcare. Imagination is not the same as fantasy. Fantasy can involve outlandish, unrealistic ways of thinking or speaking which contain unusual perspectives or sets of ideas that stimulate the mind in novel ways, but which have no real connection to 'reality' and little possibilities for bringing about change. Imagination is something quite different, something much more practical and grounded. Creative imagination is the precursor to transformative practice. In his reflections on the work of the prophet, Walter Brueggemann highlights the centrality of imagination:

> The prophet does not ask if the vision can be implemented, for questions of implementation are of no consequence until the vision can be imagined. The imagination must come before the implementation. Our culture is competent to implement almost anything and to imagine almost nothing. The same royal consciousness that makes it possible to implement anything and everything is the one that shrinks imagination because imagination is a danger. Thus every totalitarian regime is frightened of the artist. It is the vocation of the prophet to keep alive the ministry of imagination, to keep on conjuring and proposing futures alternative to the single one the king wants to urge as the only thinkable one. (Brueggemann 2001, p.45)

What Brueggemann says about the prophet can also be said about the chaplain. In a pragmatically oriented healthcare context which sometimes seems able to 'implement almost anything and to imagine almost nothing', the chaplain brings a form of transformative imagination that offers both challenge and the potential for healing. In a very real sense it is the vocation of the chaplain to keep alive the ministry of imagination, to keep on conjuring and proposing futures alternative to the single one the king '[read: the established norm] wants to urge as the only thinkable one.'

Imagination, then, is a deeply practical concept – the necessary precursor for effective transformative practices. It relates to the ways in which we conceptualize and make sense of the world, read the present situation and anticipate possible futures. To suggest that chaplaincy requires a certain form of imagination is simply to indicate that chaplains see the world slightly differently from other healthcare professions and, in imagining it differently, contribute to the healthcare imagination in important ways. The primary medium through which chaplains learn to see the world differently is story. Hospitals are deeply storied places, and chaplaincy is inevitably a narrative-based discipline. Listening to, negotiating and working with stories forms the heart of the task of healthcare chaplaincy.

The hospital as a place of stories

Human life is storied existence. In a very real sense we are the stories that we tell about ourselves and that others tell about us. To be human is to be storied; to live humanly is to be able to tell your story well and to have the right stories told about you. In rhythm with the narrative nature of humanness, healthcare is irrevocably a storied enterprise. Take, for example, the process of diagnosis in a person who has some kind of unpleasant or undesirable physical or psychological experience. They take the story of that experience and give it to the doctor, whom they hope will give clarity to the change in the plot line of their lives. The doctor then filters the story through whatever theoretical frameworks they have learned (explanatory stories about illness) and rewrites the story according to the ways in which she or he has been taught to understand the types of narrative that the person has offered. The doctor then gives the person an interpretation of the person's story, which leads to the development of a new story which in turn provides context and depth to the person's (now 'patient's', i.e. a significant change of role) new story. This new story offers fresh ways for the patient to interpret their experience and retell their story, and in so doing, to come to expect and accept certain forms of healing.

Whilst not always formally recognized, the narrative dimensions of healthcare practice run like a golden thread through all that we do. Listening to, interpreting and telling stories is the lifeblood of chaplaincy. The primary skills of the chaplain – presence, listening, empathy, spiritual discernment, working with spiritual rituals and disciplines, and so forth – are all skills designed to enable the faithful hearing of stories and the enablement of an appropriately healing response. A key task of the chaplain is to ensure that the patent's story is accurately represented in the midst of the myriad of other competing stories that comprise modern healthcare.

The hospital, then, is above all else a place of stories. It is a complex place within which stories are told, sometimes heard, always negotiated and very easily misunderstood. Whether these stories are wrapped up in diagnoses (i.e. the medical story of what is going on), in politics (the stories that administrators, managers and politicians tell about health and healthcare) or in the day-to-day stories that healthcare professionals and patients tell about health and illness, listening, hearing and responding to stories sits at the heart of the task of chaplaincy.

Negotiating and healing stories

Within such a context, a primary task of chaplaincy is narrative negotiation and narrative healing. Some of the stories that are told about health and illness are spoken in very loud voices. Stories of medication, therapy, surgery and pathology all have an inherently loud volume that can very easily overpower the personal stories of illness – the quiet voices of the ill, the dying, those losing their memories or those whose psychological distress, and the formal naming of that distress, hides and shapes the ways in which their stories are heard. People need help to negotiate the complexities of the healthcare system and to be enabled to find ways of raising up those voices that seem trivial in the eyes of the system but which are crucial for meaningful personal care.

Helping people to tell the right stories about their experiences of illness and caring is a mode of healing. By this I simply mean that in enabling people to discover new meanings in their illness stories and helping them to negotiate the complex narrative environment of healthcare contexts (helping people to tell their stories well), the chaplain encounters and encourages a profound mode of healing. Think of it in this way: The medical story lays illness out in terms of a fairly basic storyline which includes symptoms, diagnoses, treatments and desired outcomes. This basic medical plot is underpinned by another story; this story speaks of efficiency, time management, cost-effectiveness and value for money. Underneath this is yet another story that talks about how an individual is experiencing their illness, the deep phenomenological intricacies of what it means to be ill. This story is inhabited by characters who encounter fear, lost dreams, new possibilities and the need to be cared for and reoriented in the world. All of this before we even begin to contemplate the narratives of caring that each healthcare discipline brings to the patient – and in different ways! Within this complicated web of interrelated stories, the chaplain strives to listen, interpret, negotiate, advocate, clarify and answer the fundamental question: Who will help me to tell my story well?

It is in recognizing and embodying this complexity that chaplains truly find their own vital space. By bearing in their bodies and in their practices a spiritual story of illness and caregiving that seeks to reconfigure illness, from a meaningless tragedy to a meaningful and potentially transformative experience, chaplains engage in a process of radical narrative negotiation and healing that is deep, countercultural and profoundly imaginative. Chaplaincy, in this narrative mode, is really quite subversive, seeking to undermine the hopeless plots that lie behind many stories of illness and replace them with a different, fuller and more hopeful narrative. Such hopeful narratives are the essence of a refreshed healthcare imagination and the prolegomenon for effective spiritual care. Chaplains renegotiate the meanings of illness and draw attention to the fact that healing requires listening; listening requires time; time requires a different spiritual story of health and healthcare, a different kind of imagination. In this way chaplains embody the soul of healthcare systems and offer a fresh and liberated imagination.

The power of case studies:
Thick and thin descriptions

All of this brings us to the deep and transformative power that is revealed in the types of case studies that are offered in this book. *Illnesses have complex meanings and caring is a multidimensional task.* Experiencing illness and caring for people encountering illness is not a thin biomedical practice that can be done apart from the uniqueness of the individual; rather, such things are rich, deep and deeply personal experiences that occur within the lives of unique individuals who reside within communities that care. If we are to understand the experience of illness and what it means to care for people who are ill, we need rich and thick descriptions. Such things as diagnoses, case notes and casual conversations around interpersonal encounters can be thin and instrumental. Case studies are inevitably thick descriptions of human experience that help us to engage at a deep level with the 'hidden' experiences of illness and caring.

The anthropologist Clifford Geertz talks about the idea of thick and thin descriptions (Geertz 1973). The task of the anthropologist, Geertz insists, is to explore culture through the process of providing rich and thick descriptions of what is going on. A thick description tries to capture the complex dynamics of any given situation – its symbols, perspectives, the meanings that are hidden to outsiders, the boundaries of that which is plausible and that which is not – and to present them in a way that helps the reader to fully understand the situation, experience or context. A thin description, on the other hand, is a simple, factual account without any interpretation and without any attempt to get to grips with the complexities of situations and human beings within those situations. The problem with thin descriptions is not simply that they are inadequate, but that they are actually misleading. Bald facts without context or interpretation are only facts in a minimal sense. It is only really when we get into the thickness of a situation or experience that we discover what it truly is. This is precisely what case studies allow us to do: get into the thick of it! They grab our attention and pull us into the intricate complexity of the experience of being ill and receiving care. Case study work enables chaplains to see things that other approaches simply do not enable them to see. They help to develop a certain kind of imagination that is central to what chaplains are and what they do.

Conclusion: Thickening our imagination

A case study approach offers chaplains unique opportunities to contribute creatively to the development of the healthcare imagination. Case studies move chaplaincy away from the temptation to become evidence-based in ways that are thin, obvious and conformist, and to open up a space for an approach that is original, necessary, imaginative and truly person centred. The cases laid out in this book are fine examples of what chaplains do and why they do it; they show quite clearly why it is really unimaginable to have a healthcare system that does not include the richness of perception and the depth of understanding that chaplaincy brings. Of course, sadly, for many it *is* imaginable that we could have healthcare without chaplains. But that is only because some people lack the kind of imagination that is necessary to care well.

References

Brueggemann, W. (2001) *The Prophetic Imagination* (2nd edn). Minneapolis, MN: Augsburg Fortress.

Geertz, C. (1973) 'Thick description: Toward an interpretive theory of culture.' In C. Geertz (ed) *The Interpretation of Cultures: Selected Essays*. New York, NY: Basic Books, 3–30.

Contributors

Alister W. Bull, BD, Dip Min, MTh, PhD, was for 12 years NHS Healthcare Chaplain at Yorkhill Children's Hospital, Glasgow and lead chaplain at Glasgow Royal Infirmary, UK. He now works for the Church of Scotland as Secretary to the Mission and Discipleship Council.

Sian Cotton, PhD, a health psychologist, is the Director of the Center for Integrative Health and Wellness and UC Health Integrative Medicine at the University of Cincinnati, USA. She regularly teaches and conducts mixed-methods research on complementary/integrative health approaches including mind-body therapies, mindfulness, religion/ spirituality, coping with chronic illness and quality of life.

George Fitchett, DMin, PhD, is Professor and Director of Research, Department of Religion, Health and Human Values, Rush University Medical Center, Chicago, Illinois, USA. Trained as a chaplain and a researcher (epidemiology), he leads a program of research focused on the role of religion/spirituality in coping with illness and the development of a research-informed approach to chaplaincy care.

Graeme D. Gibbons, DMin, BA, BD, Grad Dip Psych, is an ordained minister of the Uniting Church in Australia, and accredited Clinical Pastoral Educator by the Association of Supervised Pastoral Education in Australia. As a registered psychologist he conducts a private practice in psychotherapy and supervision from a psychoanalytical self-psychology and process theology perspective.

Daniel H. Grossoehme, DMin, BCC, is an Associate Professor of Pediatrics (Division of Pulmonary Medicine) at Cincinnati Children's Hospital Medical Center and Staff Chaplain III (Department of Pastoral

Care). An Episcopal priest and a pediatric chaplain for over 20 years, he currently divides his time between clinical chaplaincy and health outcomes research.

Alice A. Hildebrand, MDiv, BCC, is the Women's and Children's Service Line Chaplain at Barbara Bush Children's Hospital of Maine Medical Center, Portland, Maine, USA. She holds an MDiv from Bangor Theological Seminary and is Board Certified by the Association of Professional Chaplains. She is ordained in the United Church of Christ.

Jim Huth, PhD, is a spiritual care provider at Sunnybrook Veterans Centre, Toronto, Canada. He is a specialist with the Canadian Association for Spiritual Care and the vice-chair of its national ethics committee. He is a lecturer (status-only) with the Department of Occupational Therapy and Occupational Sciences, University of Toronto.

Warren Kinghorn, MD, ThD, is Assistant Professor of Psychiatry and Pastoral and Moral Theology at Duke University Medical Center and Duke Divinity School, and a staff psychiatrist at the Durham VA Medical Center, North Carolina, USA. His research explores the role of religious communities in the care of people with mental health problems.

David B. McCurdy, DMin, BCC, is an adjunct faculty member in Religious Studies at Elmhurst College, Illinois, USA. Recently retired from Advocate Health Care, he was a senior ethics consultant and Director of Organizational Ethics at Advocate. He is a board certified chaplain (APC) and a certified supervisor of clinical pastoral education (ACPE).

David Mitchell, BD, Dip P Theo, MSc, PG Cert, TLHE, is programme leader for Postgraduate Education in Healthcare Chaplaincy at the University of Glasgow, UK. He serves as an executive member of the UK Board of Healthcare Chaplaincy with a particular focus on standards, capabilities and competences for healthcare chaplains.

Steve Nolan, PhD, has been chaplain at Princess Alice Hospice, Esher, UK, since 2004. He holds a PhD from the University of Manchester and is dual qualified as a BACP accredited counsellor/psychotherapist. Previous publications include *Spiritual Care at the End of Life: The Chaplain as a 'Hopeful Presence'* (2012).

Barbara Pesut, PhD, RN, is Canada Research Chair in Health, Ethics and Diversity. Associate Professor, School of Nursing, University of British Columbia, Okanagan, she researches improvements in end-of-life care for people at risk of health disparities. Projects explore healthcare implications of changing understandings of spirituality, negotiating spiritual/religious differences and spiritual care education.

Katherine M. Piderman, PhD, BCC, is a staff chaplain at Mayo Clinic, Rochester, Minnesota, USA. Ministering to patients and their loved ones during times of crisis, treatment and transition, she also coordinates and contributes to clinically related spiritual research with several patient populations, working closely with the healthcare team to support the best of outcomes.

Christina M. Puchalski, MD, is a professor of Medicine and Health Sciences at the George Washington University School of Medicine, Washington DC, where she founded and directs the George Washington Institute for Spirituality and Health (GWish). She developed the FICA spiritual assessment tool, and her books include *Time for Listening and Caring: Spirituality and the Care of the Seriously Ill and Dying* (2006) and the co-edited *Oxford Textbook of Spirituality in Healthcare* (2012).

Rosie Ratcliffe, PhD, is Trust Chaplain and Mental Health Lead at Imperial College Healthcare NHS Trust, London. She completed a Masters at Kings College, London, before ordination in 2001, and worked in mental health chaplaincy for 14 years, while lecturing in biblical studies at King's College where she completed a PhD. Her publications are in biblical studies and chaplaincy.

Nina Redl, BCC, currently works at Bryan Medical Center, Lincoln, Nebraska, USA, where she specializes in palliative oncology, trauma and intensive care chaplaincy for patients of all ages. She has worked as a chaplain in the USA, Germany and the Middle East.

Wes Roberts, MTS, BRE, is a chaplain in the Veterans Centre at Sunnybrook Health Sciences Centre of Toronto specializing in dementia care, where his contributions include co-facilitating the Accreditation Canada Leading Practice (2010) Partners in Veterans Care initiative. He holds advanced chaplaincy standing with the Canadian Association for Spiritual Care and is ordained with The Christian and Missionary Alliance in Canada.

Christopher Swift, PhD, is Head of Chaplaincy Services at the Leeds Teaching Hospitals NHS Trust, one of England's largest acute hospital trusts, and Visiting Research Fellow at the University of Leeds. He has active research interests in ethnography and chaplaincy, and has written extensively on issues relating to chaplaincy provision, notably *Hospital Chaplaincy in the Twenty-first Century* (2014).

John Swinton, PhD, BD, RNM, RNHD, is Professor in Practical Theology and Pastoral Care in the School of Divinity, Religious Studies and Philosophy at the University of Aberdeen, UK. He has a background in nursing and healthcare chaplaincy and has researched and published extensively within the areas of practical theology, mental health, spirituality and human well-being, and the theology of disability.

Richard C. Weyls, MDiv, STL, BCC is a staff chaplain on the Palliative Care Consult Team, Swedish Health Systems, Seattle, Washington, USA. An ordained minister, endorsed for chaplaincy by the Episcopal Church USA and board certified with the Association of Professional Chaplains, he works in the acute-care setting with a concentration in palliative and critical care.

Angelika A. Zollfrank, BCC, ACPE, formerly Clinical Pastoral Educator and inpatient psychiatric chaplain, Massachusetts General Hospital, Boston, USA; now Coordinator of Pastoral Education and medical unit chaplain, Yale New Haven Hospital, Connecticut, USA. A Clinical Pastoral Education Supervisor with the Association for Clinical Pastoral Education, she is also a licensed systems-centered practitioner (SCTRI).

Index